PRAISE FOR

HOW MUCH DOES A ZEBRA WEIGH?

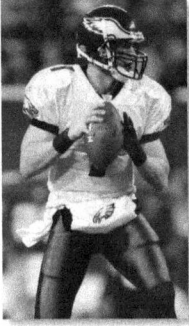

"The knowledge contained in this book is what separates the average athlete from the champion. I strive to be the best at everything I do. I realize that in wanting to be the best, I have to be willing to sacrifice and work. Perfection, dominance, excellence, and finishing are what I look to as an end result or accomplishment for my hard work and dedication. Whether I attain these goals depends upon my own attitude and my vision as to what I want to achieve on a daily basis. I know that when I train with Kyle, the emphasis is going to be a high-intensity, get-after-it mentality that I like to call organized chaos. We have a plan, a purpose, and the goal is to push myself beyond a level that I could ever reach when training on my own. Thanks, Kyle, for always pushing me to that championship level that I expect from myself."

— Jeff Garcia, NFL Quarterback with the Houston Texans, seventeen-year professional career

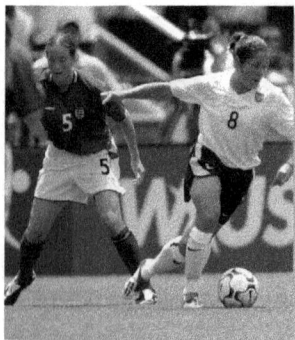

"Never give up! During my twelve-year career with the U.S. Women's National Team, I had many roles. I was a starter, I was dubbed the "super sub," and I was even cut from the team. It would have been easy to give up and walk away, but I chose to fight. In 1996, I was cut from the Olympic team, but instead of giving up, I worked twice as hard and eventually not only earned a spot on the roster of sixteen to represent the U.S. at the Atlanta Olympics, but also was a starter and finished the tournament as the leading scorer. You have to always believe in yourself and learn to embrace the challenge. When things are hard, you learn to appreciate and enjoy the successes even more! The World Championship and the gold medals are cherished, but what I cherish more are the friends I made along the way and the life lessons I was able to extract from the wins as well as the challenges. *How Much Does A Zebra Weigh?* is all about challenging yourself to achieve your true potential."

— Shannon Mac Millan, U.S. Olympic Gold Medalist, Women's Soccer, 1999 Women's World Cup Champion, twelve-year career with U.S. Women's National Team, with 176 games, 1995 Hermann Trophy Winner, Best Female Collegiate Soccer Player

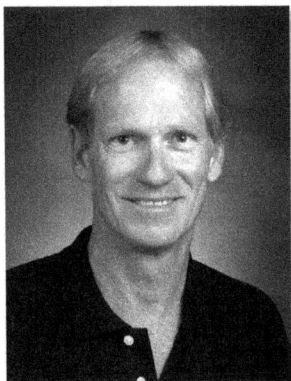

"One of the best ways to combat childhood obesity is by limiting or eliminating processed foods, refined grains and sugars and replacing them with fresh fruits, vegetables, fresh meat, poultry and seafood. *How Much Does A Zebra Weigh?*'s focus on Paleolithic nutrition will help you take the first step for better health and freedom from obesity."

— Dr. Loren Cordain, Ph.D., Professor, Department of Health and Exercise Science at Colorado State University, author of the bestselling books *The Paleo Diet*, *The Paleo Diet Cookbook* and *The Paleo Answer*.

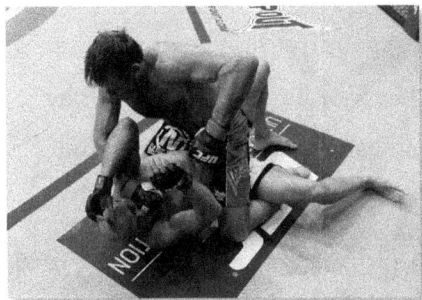

"As in life, martial arts and fighting are filled with numerous obstacles. The ups are great, but the downs can be devastating. Every fighter goes through these to some extent or another. Working through these downs is what builds character and discipline. The secrets in *How Much Does A Zebra Weigh?* will empower you to build your self-confidence so you can conquer any obstacle."

— Stephan "The American Psycho" Bonnar
Ultimate Fighting Championships (UFC) Light Heavyweight Fighter
The Ultimate Fighter Season 1 Finalist

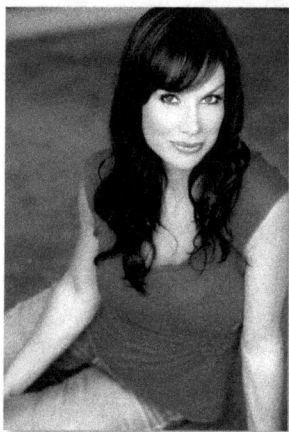

"As a working mother of three with a new walker, I have to say that time is my most important asset. Kyle's fitness and nutrition tips in this book keep my health and fitness on the A-list so I can continue to work in Hollywood and have energy left for my family. I get results faster and better than anyone I have worked with in the past."

— Debbe Dunning, Actress/Mother, Heidi, the Tool Time Girl from *Home Improvement*

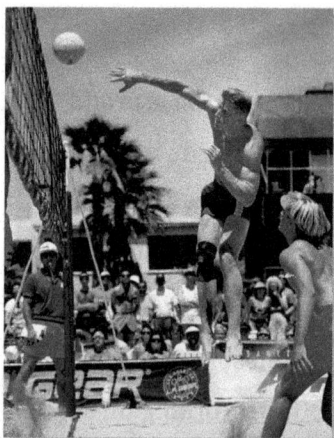

"Now that I've hit fifty, it is not about going for the gold anymore. It's about staying pain-free and healthy. Based on what Kyle has taught me and the principles in this book, my workouts are fun and interesting and keep me going as a father and businessman so I can go for the gold in the rest of my life."

— Steve Timmons, Three-Time Gold Medalist, Volleyball

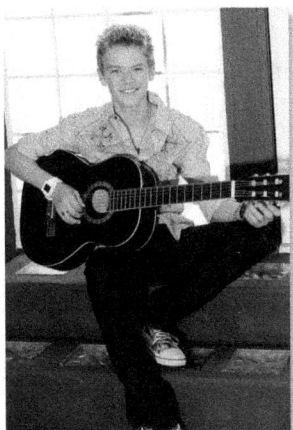

"Learning how to eat healthy and live a balanced lifestyle have been very important tools for me becoming successful as a young actor. I enjoy cooking healthy meals. Kyle Brown's *How Much Does A Zebra Weigh?* will teach you how to achieve your potential and eat delicious, healthy food the way nature intended. These concepts and tips are so important and will stay with me for my life's journey! Dream big!"

— Kenton Duty, Actor Disney Channel's *Shake It Up!* and ABC's *Lost*

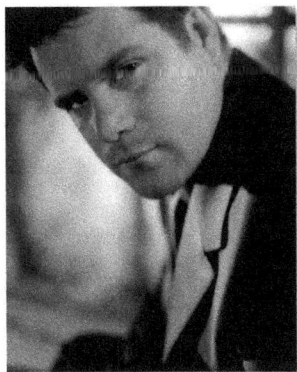

"The most important lesson that people take away from one of the films I'm known for, *Rudy,* is that you should never accept the limitations that others put on you. It is so important to decide for yourself what you are capable of. You should dream big and never give up. No matter how big or small you are, ya gotta have guts and be tough and stubborn to get where you are going. And here's a secret: in a weird way, these qualities can actually be fun!"

— Sean Astin, Actor, Director, Producer, Mikey Walsh in *The Goonies*, Rudy in *Rudy*, and Samwise Gamgee in *The Lord of the Rings* trilogy

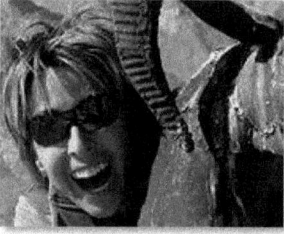

"Living the life of a champion is about being healthy in mind and body and never underestimating yourself. *How Much Does A Zebra Weigh?* will help you live your best life possible."

— Siri Lindley, Triathlon World Champion and Former World #1. Coach of Champions: Kona Ironman, World Champion 2010 and 70.3, and Mirinda Carfrae, World Champion 2007. Coach of Olympic Triathlon Medalists (Susan Williams, USA, 2004), National Champions, World Number-ones and consistent winners. Owner, Sirius Athletes, LLC.

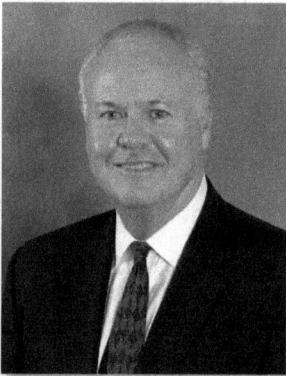

"Conquering the bullying crisis requires empathy, a healthy dialogue, and a proactive approach. *How Much Does A Zebra Weigh?* provides excellent tools for empowering today's youth to achieve their potential, gain confidence, and become tomorrow's leaders."

—Tom Turner, Chairman of the National Conflict Resolution Center, Managing Partner at Procopio, Cory, Hargreaves & Savitch LLP

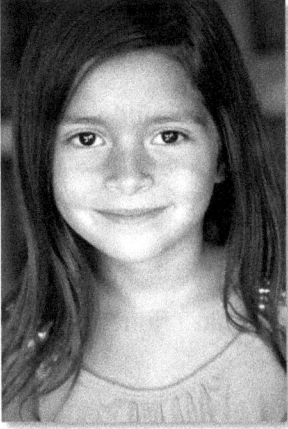

"Just like you'll learn in this book, I will always hold my hand out to pick someone up; I will never be the one to push someone down!"

— Alexys Nycole Sanchez, Actress Becky in Adam Sandler's movie *Grown Ups*, Winner 2011 MTV Movie Award's Best Line in a Movie: "I want to get chocolate wasted!"

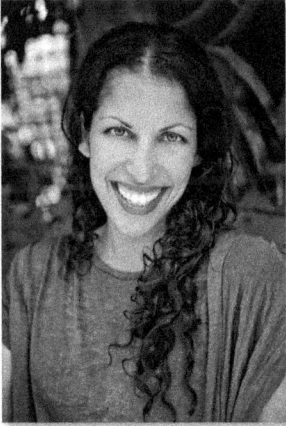

"As a pediatrician, every day I see that kids who develop healthy nutrition and lifestyle habits when they are young are setting themselves up for success. *How Much Does A Zebra Weigh?* offers practical, easy-to-understand tools that you can apply and start improving your quality of life right away!"

— Dr. Shakha Gillin, Pediatrician

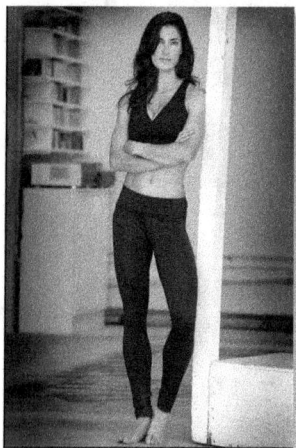

"What you eat before and after you work out is just as important as what you do during your workout. You wouldn't fuel a Ferrari with regular gas, right? *How Much Does A Zebra Weigh?* will take your health and fitness to celebrity status!"
— Natasha Kufa, Personal Trainer to the Stars

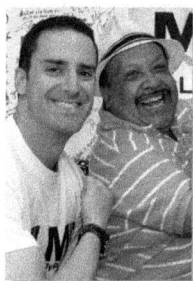

"As you will learn in this book, no matter what anyone says, you have the power do anything and be anything! Stay positive, work hard and keep a sense of humor!"
— Chuy Bravo, Chelsea Handler's sidekick on E!'s #1 rated show *Chelsea Lately*, actor in *Austin Powers 3: Goldmember, The Rundown*, and *Pirates of the Caribbean: At World's End*

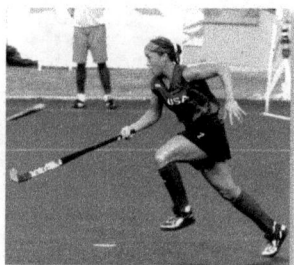

"I played team sports from the time I was five years old and had a lot of coaches. The most important thing I learned is to never give your power away! But how do you do that, you ask? Preparation! You need confidence in sports and life, and true confidence comes from a deep-rooted belief in yourself, not

from anything anyone ever says to you. Sometimes we might have bullies, coaches, teachers, friends, or parents telling us we aren't any good, but they don't know you! Only you know what kind of effort you put forth. If you try your hardest and fail, which you will sometimes, you should feel good about it. Sure, it's not fun to lose, but losing is a part of sports and life. You don't always get to win, but you do get to control exactly how much effort you put in. Sure, it feels great when a coach tells you, 'Good job.' But you shouldn't start playing badly just because the coach begins yelling at you. That's giving them your power. Hear their words but don't let them affect your play. Listen and learn and believe in yourself because you have prepared. *How Much Does A Zebra Weigh?* will show you that if you do your best, work your hardest, pay attention, eat well, and are thoughtful, you have every right to be confident."
— Kristen Fillat, 1996 U.S. Olympian, Field Hockey, Three-Time World Cup Team, Three-Time Pan American Team, Founder/CEO of the GoodOnYa Bar & Café

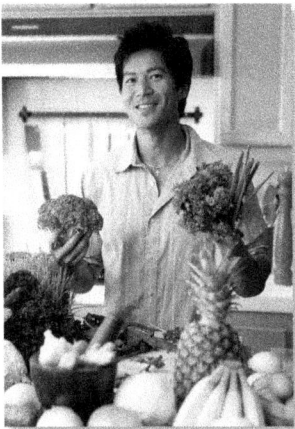

"Knowing where your food comes from, how to prepare it in the most nutritious way, and being in tune with what your body needs is one of the keys to living a healthy lifestyle. *How Much Does A Zebra Weigh?* will show you how easy it is to start making a change today!"
— Chef Minh Nguyen, Fitness Nutrition Chef

HOW MUCH

DOES A

ZEBRA WEIGH?

Written by: Kyle Brown

Contributors: Chef Minh Nguyen, Dave Gleason, and Darren Rudsinski

Cover Design and Layout: Brian McCurdy

Illustrator: Chris Branham

Editors: Tricia Rott and Michelle Dotter

Photographer: Barry Wayne

Publisher's Disclaimer

The material in this book is for informational purposes only. As each individual's situation is unique, you should consult a health care provider before undertaking the diet, exercise, and lifestyle techniques described in this book. The author and publisher expressly disclaim responsibility for any adverse effects that may result from the use or application of the information contained in this book.

Acknowledgements

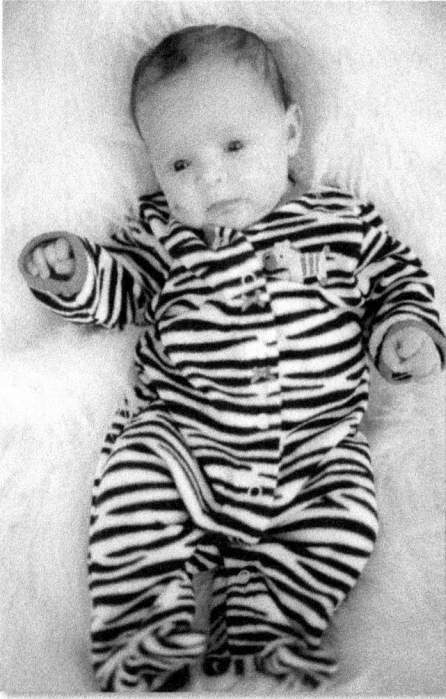

This book is dedicated to all of the kids around the world who are ready to empower themselves with the knowledge presented here and to develop the skills that will enable them to be champions for the rest of their lives.

A big thank-you to all of the athletes, celebrities, corporations, police officers, sheriffs, teachers, counselors and individuals who have chosen to stand up as role models and help us teach kids how to empower themselves to reach their true potential.

I dedicate this book to my beautiful, loving and supportive wife, Sarah, and my new baby, Ava. Hope for my children's future is why I wrote this book and dedicated myself to fighting childhood obesity. Also to my loving parents, Bob and Sherry Brown, and my siblings, Andy, Cameron and Vanessa, and my extended family; my successful family (in all senses of the word) has always motivated me to strive to achieve greatness and to put family first. To my puppies MJ and Ahava, who taught me to study animals to learn how to eat and exercise properly and to love unconditionally. And finally, to my friends, who gave me the support network to become a champion.

Table of Contents

fast food! Best of all, you'll have a step-by-step game plan in the Strive 4 Fitness® 21-day game to get started today!

How to execute your plan of action and achieve your goals

Your kick-start to transform the way you look, feel, and think in just 21 days

Introduction: The Champion Lifestyle

Are you ready to turn your dreams into a reality? Now is your time!

"As long as you keep moving forward, no matter how many people keep pushing you backward, you'll keep moving forward."
— Kyle Brown

This book will be the best class you've ever taken. You'll want to keep it for a lifetime and revisit it regularly for healthy lifestyle secrets that only world-class athletes and highly educated natural health aficionados know.

In many classes, your focus is on memorizing information to make a grade and then moving forward with your education. The information gets crammed into your brain for a test and then vanishes once the exam is over. The best thing about this class is that there are no grades and no one is judging you! It's more than just one class; it's a variety of classes that all combine to transform you into a better, more well-rounded person. And unlike many classes in school, you won't struggle to see how it applies to your life. You'll get out of it what you put into it. Best of all, you can start applying what you learn today! Like anything else in life, the more effort you put into learning how to apply the information in this book, the more success you'll achieve. Anything in life worth having requires hard work and sacrifice.

I am not here to tell you what to do or how to live your life. I am here as your ally, your friend, your mentor—a guy with a wealth of experience and information who can help you achieve the healthy mind, body and habits that will enable you to build the successful life you've always wanted.

The power to be a champion is within you. But first you need to understand what being a champion really means.

Being a true champion is not about how many honors, accolades or trophies you earn. It's not about how much money you make or how popular you are. It's about living a life of self-worth and leaving behind a better legacy. Champions are admired by their community for their hard work. Champions feel it's their civic responsibility to help make the world a better place, now and for future generations. They think globally but act locally. They are also champions of a cause, such as putting a stop to the challenges harming today's youth, like childhood obesity and bullying. Champions think beyond themselves and figure out how they can improve their communities as a whole.

After looking at the root causes of problems like lack of focus in school, kids without a clear direction, and a lack of contribution by adults to their communities, I have learned that we need to start young and teach kids how to set goals, stick to them and work hard to succeed in life.

How Much Does A Zebra Weigh? **promotes the progressive concept that anyone who strives to better him or herself physically, mentally and emotionally is an athlete. An athlete is someone who strives to live the highest quality of life possible.**

You're not only an athlete if you play traditional sports—anyone who challenges himself or herself to participate in theatre, dance, choir, public speaking or any other activity that involves becoming a more well-rounded, holistic person is an athlete.

As an athlete or a leader in your school, once you've learned the secrets of champions and begun applying them to your life, you'll have both the ability and the responsibility to use these secrets to help others. The time to act is now. By living the life of a champion and taking just one person who's less fortunate than you under your wing, you can take a significant step toward making the world a better place. A little help goes a long way. And please note that the key to combating the crises that are plaguing today's youth is empathy. Empathy is the ability to understand and share another person's feelings. The first step to becoming empathetic is communication. Listen to and communicate with others in your community who need your help, and then give back by offering your talents, your passions and your time. Start small by asking other kids how they are doing and really listening to the answer. Offer an empathetic ear or lend a hand. You can make a powerful impact by just listening to and helping one person improve their quality of life.

PART 1:

Secrets to

Becoming

Your Best You

Chapter 1:

Enjoy the Ride

Think, feel, believe and project the person you wish to be

Imagine yourself out in the park, with a basketball in hand, playing an impromptu game with friends. You're laughing, smiling, and having a good time—not a care in the world. It's like a form of Tai Chi, meditation in motion.

When do the best athletes in nearly every sport have their best performances? When they're completely in the moment, acting like a kid, pressure-free, enjoying the process. They're not focusing on the mechanics or the pressure of the game. They're having fun and everything simply gels. They're laughing, they're smiling—they're remembering why they started playing that sport in the first place.

This philosophy applies to anyone trying to live a healthy and fit lifestyle. Just like when you are on a road trip with your family, you need to enjoy the ride instead of whining, "Are we there yet?" Every aspect of your training and nutrition should feel this way. You eat healthy because it makes you feel good. The food tastes delicious, and when you're done eating you feel full and satisfied, your energy renewed. You're excited to walk into the gym and lift weights because it makes you feel strong. You're amped to go to practice because it makes you better at the game you love. You drink water because you feel healthy and energized. The key is to get to the why.

When you were a really young kid, "Why?" was most likely your favorite question. I'm sure you constantly asked your friends and family why something was the way it was and "Because I said so" was never a good enough answer. The answer to "why" is your purpose. It's the reason behind your actions, your effort, and your sacrifice. It's the reason you do what you do. And your "why" may be different from my "why" or from your friends' or family's "why." One of the big mistakes young athletes make is that their initial "why" gets replaced by the fantasy of becoming rich and famous. Those are potential side benefits of achieving your goals but should not be the reason you're striving for them in the first place. Your "why" should be based around improving your quality of life.

You need to focus on enjoying the ride. These twelve secrets are not a checklist, but a journey. The goal is not to memorize the secrets in this book but to live and breathe them, and for them to become part of your personal culture. These secrets should eventually become part of who you are at the core. Not approaching your goals in this manner is the problem of nearly every adult. They know what they do and focus on learning how to do what they do, but they forget their purpose. For example, I've seen many athletes do whatever it takes to become a professional athlete. Yet of these select few who actually make it, the overwhelming majority crash and burn once they get there. This phenomenon happens partially because they don't set goals for what they're going to do once they become a professional, but mostly because their "why" has become tainted in the process. They've lost their love for the game and stopped striving for greatness. The goal is to be happy but not content. You should always strive to be the best you can be.

And it's not just athletes. I've also seen this happen with people who are trying to lose weight or gain muscle. They focus all their energy on reaching a particular number on their scale and follow an approach based solely on temporary sacrifice. As soon as they reach their scale weight goal, they typically start eating poorly again and stop exercising as frequently. It's disastrous! Weight loss has little to do with willpower. It's about developing a mindset and enriching yourself with proper information.

Many teens trying to get fit put forth a ton of effort but are misguided by poor information. Instead, you need a game plan that helps create healthy habits and daily rituals that will get you to the top and keep you on top. And the process needs to be fun rather than a miserable sacrifice. Quick fixes are not acceptable, as they are inconsistent with long-term change. Thinking "the diet starts tomorrow" is setting yourself up for failure. Instead, use my motto: "The healthy lifestyle starts now." Do this for your own reasons, your own "why" for wanting to improve your quality of life today. And always remember: enjoy the ride, as it will make you emotionally fit and psychologically strong.

Key takeaways from this chapter:

- When do the best athletes in nearly every sport have their best performances? When they're completely in the moment, acting like a kid, pressure-free, enjoying the process.

- The key is to get to the "why." The answer to "why" is your purpose. It's the reason behind your actions, your effort, and your sacrifice.
- One of the big mistakes many teens make is that their initial "why" gets replaced by the fantasy of becoming rich and famous.
- Weight loss has little to do with willpower. It's about developing a mindset and enriching yourself with proper information.

Chapter 2

The Holistic Approach of a True Champion

Practice doesn't end when you leave the field—it's just beginning

You have their posters on your wall; you pretend to be them as you practice your favorite sport; you dream one day to walk in their footsteps, and you idolize them as real-life superheroes because they rise above the rest. Champion athletes like Michael Jordan, Lance Armstrong, Peyton Manning, Michael Phelps, Bo Jackson, and Georges St-Pierre all share a common secret. In addition to their natural talent, they have solid discipline and a strong work ethic that elevates them to champion status. They are the first ones to arrive at practice and the last ones to leave. Moreover, practice doesn't end when they leave the field; it's just beginning. With the help of a team of experts, they've mastered all of the secrets of a true champion: nutrition, supplementation, exercise, flexibility, quality sleep, stress management, positive mental attitude, the I.F. (Internal Fortitude) factor, and keeping it fun. They may have different philosophies about each of these elements, but bottom line, they all constantly work to fine-tune them.

When I played high school sports, the coaching focus was on giving 110% effort during practice. Those who put forth the most effort were praised for their hustle and those who lagged behind were often ridiculed for their lack of energy or focus. Coaches put all of their effort into detailed instruction of that particular sport's mechanics, rules, game strategy, and teamwork. Yet once practice ended, so did the coaching. In any of the sports I played—even through college and beyond—there was no game plan to cover the healthy lifestyle disciplines required to perform at the highest level. Resistance training was encouraged, but things like sport-specific exercise, rest/recovery protocols, and pre- and post-workout nutrition were never addressed. Now, I don't blame the coaches for this failure, as these other disciplines are not their forte. They are trained to coach the particular skill set of that sport and motivate and organize the athletes. Unfortunately, this is where the scope of practice ends. They simply don't have the time or the resources to address all of the elements of champions.

A holistic lifestyle approach to health and fitness is cutting-edge information that most athletes, including professional athletes in every sport, aren't taught. Only elite athletes understand the key to unlocking their true athletic potential is addressing all of these elements and making them a priority. They understand that it's not only about hard work, but about working smart and keeping it fun. They are fortunate to see the big picture.

Champions surround themselves with a team of professionals. A champion racing team has an entire pit crew working in unity to ensure their high-performance car is running optimally, from monitoring the fuel, oil, and tire pressure to making wedge adjustments that give their driver the competitive edge in a high-tech sport. If there is any indication that something is wrong, the driver immediately brings the car in to the pit crew for evaluation.

The human body is a vastly more complex machine, far more valuable, and requires much more preventative maintenance. Yet unlike the racecar driver, who focuses on preventative maintenance, the typical teen only focuses on issues when they arise. The typical teen only sees a doctor when they're sick, a dentist when they have a toothache, an optometrist when their vision needs to be checked, and a physical therapist when they need injury rehabilitation. Teens all know they are not experts in these fields, so they seek the guidance of a professional. Yet they seem to think they can simply read a fitness magazine, take one nutrition class, watch a movie, or talk to their friends, coaches, or parents to become experts in nutrition and fitness!

The group of athletes who tend to miss the boat the most are those who are naturally gifted in sports. They are the ones who are able to excel at a sport while in junior high and high school without putting in the hard work off the field. They tend to think, "I'm one of the best players on the team and I look good, so none of this applies to me." This is a common misconception that leads to these athletes peaking in high school. They do not develop the lifestyle skills that will carry them into college and potentially professional sports, let alone a long and vibrant life. These are the kids who show up to their ten-year high school reunion thirty pounds overweight, living a sedentary, unhealthy life, clueless about the fundamental lifestyle habits required to keep fit, athletic, and healthy.

Let's face it: depending on the sport (baseball, basketball, soccer or football), between 3% and 6.1% of high school athletes play NCAA college sports. Between 1% and 9.4% of NCAA athletes play professional sports. And only 0.02 to 0.45% of high school athletes go straight to the pros. [1] Even if you are one of the few athletes who becomes a professional, 78% of NFL players go bankrupt within two years of retirement and 60% of NBA players go bankrupt within five years of retirement. [2] The average NFL player's career is only three years, compared to five years in the NBA and NHL and 5.6 years in the MLB. [3] Since the average professional athlete retires in their mid-to-late twenties, that leaves these athletes with three-quarters of their lives left to live. They will need to become professionals at something else after their sports careers come to an end. Therefore, the best investment you can make for your long-term vitality is developing the skill sets that will make you a champion in every facet of your life.

High school is about creating the habits and rituals that will help you in the long term, as life is a marathon, not a sprint. These physical, mental, and emotional tools will help you look better, feel better, have more energy, and most importantly perform better all around. This section will give you a glimpse into what the best of the best athletes do that takes them far beyond the playing field into a lifestyle of fitness, health, and happiness—and gives them an unseen edge over the competition. While I can't make these changes for you, I can give you the resources to evoke the changes within yourself.

Key takeaways from this chapter:

- In addition to their natural talent, the best of the best athletes in the world have solid discipline and a strong work ethic that elevates them to champion status.

- With the help of a team of experts, world-class athletes have mastered all of the secrets of a true champion: nutrition, supplementation, exercise, flexibility, quality sleep, stress management, positive mental attitude, the I.F. (Internal Fortitude) factor, and keeping it fun.

- The best investment you can make for your long-term vitality is developing the skill sets that will make you a champion in every facet of your life.

- High school is about creating the habits and rituals that will help you in the long term, as life is a marathon, not a sprint.

Chapter 3

Stop Counting Calories—It's Making You Fat and Weak!
Nutritional quality trumps nutritional quantity

Your body becomes what you eat. Nutrition is your foundation. It's your fuel. It affects everything from your health and energy levels to your self-image, how you look and feel, and your athletic performance. I've had countless young athletes come see me with goals of jumping higher, running faster, or improving their agility. But when I perform a body composition analysis, they register as clinically obese. And you wouldn't guess it by looking at them in street clothes. Skinny arms and legs and baggy clothes can easily hide a tire around the midsection. Once these young athletes changed their nutrition and shed the excess body fat, they were able to achieve all of their goals. Want proof? Step onto a basketball court and time yourself running from one baseline of the court to the other. Then time yourself running suicide drills. (Suicide drills are drills run on a basketball court to increase your court speed and agility). Lastly, measure your vertical jump with a vertical jump tester. Now, imagine packing your backpack with all of your heaviest textbooks and running through this same series of tests. Do you think your numbers would be worse? Of course they would.

This is the roadblock that every overweight youth faces every time they step onto the field, and it can be overcome by simply addressing all of the elements of a healthy lifestyle.

The first secret is to stop counting calories—it's making you fat and weak! And if being overweight is not an issue for you, bad nutrition is still affecting your energy levels, your athletic performance, your ability to perform in school, and your overall health. You need to become aware that nutritional quality is more important than nutritional quantity. Nutritional quality refers to the source of the food that you eat. Nutritional quantity refers to the calorie count and macronutrient percentages (grams of protein, carbohydrate, and fat) of the foods that you eat. This secret goes against everything that mainstream America preaches, as most diets are based on depriving yourself of calories and nutrients. They rely on the equation called the law of thermodynamics, which states that if you burn more calories than you consume you will lose weight, and conversely, if you consume more calories than you burn, you will gain weight. Well, who said anything about losing weight? Your goals are to sculpt a lean and fit body by maintaining or gaining lean muscle mass while losing body fat—not scale weight. Moreover, if you're an athlete, your objective is to perform better. When you consume a low-nutrient, low-calorie diet, you will most likely initially lose weight, but that weight will be primarily in the form of water and lean muscle tissue, not body fat. Rather than helping your performance as an athlete, this will actually hinder it.

I am not saying that portion control isn't important, but focusing primarily on caloric restriction isn't working in the long term for American adults, nor is it ideal for you. According to the National Institute of Health, 98% of all Americans who lose weight gain it back, and then some, within five years. Humans are the only animals that are consistently sick and fat, and yet we are the only animals who count calories. No other animal in the animal kingdom has any idea what a calorie is. In fact, most humans have no idea what a calorie is, either.

If you were to walk into a health club, how many people in there would admit to counting calories? Probably the majority of members. According to the International Food Information Council Foundation's 2010 Food and Health Survey, 75% of Americans attempt to keep track of the calories they consume. Yet only 12% can accurately estimate the number of calories they should consume in a day based on their age, height, weight, and physical activity. Of those who say they are trying to lose or maintain weight, only 19% say they are keeping track of calories. Additionally, almost half of Americans do not know how many calories they burn in a day (43%) or offer inaccurate estimates (35% say one thousand calories or less). When it comes to calories consumed versus calories burned, most Americans (58%) do not make an effort to balance the two.

How many Americans know what a calorie is? Probably very few. The Merriam-Webster dictionary defines a calorie as "the amount of heat required at a pressure of one atmosphere to raise the temperature of one gram of water one degree Celsius." Does it really make sense that you should be thinking about all of this every time you are deciding what to eat? Instead, you should be focusing on the quality of the nutrients that you eat.

Nature made it easy for us to know what to eat. Our access to food and on-the-go lifestyle demands have messed it up. To correct this problem, we need to start by going back to our hunter/gatherer roots and Paleolithic nutrition. According to the man at the forefront of Paleolithic nutrition research, Dr. Loren Cordain, Paleolithic nutrition is a way of looking at our nutritional needs as a product of a multimillion year evolutionary process. As our DNA has shifted less than 1% from our Paleolithic ancestors, we are still physiologically constructed to eat this diet 2.5 million years later,. We haven't had enough time to genetically adapt ourselves to the agricultural changes of the last 10,000 years, let alone the last 100 years of refining. [4] Paleolithic nutrition basically consists of consuming lean meats and fish (from animals that eat what they are supposed to), seasonal vegetables, small amounts of fruits, nuts and seeds, and healthy oils.

The following is a comparison chart of how we used to eat in Paleolithic times versus the Standard American Diet.

Paleolithic Diet	Modern/Standard American Diet
2.5 million years (1% shift in DNA)	10,000 years into last 100 years of refining
90% of carbohydrates consumed were derived from Fruits and Vegetables	Carbohydrates consumed are primarily in the form of Grains and Refined Sugars
1-2% Simple Sugars	23% Fruits and Vegetables
	18-20% Simple Sugars

Protein	Protein
LOW in Saturated Fat	HIGH in Saturated Fat
LOW Sodium and NO Chemical Residues	HIGH Sodium with 600 Residues
Less Total Fat	More Total Fat
3-4% Game Animal Fat	20-25% Domestic Animal Fat
2x as much Unsaturated Fat	2.5x as much Saturated Fat
Unsaturated Fat to Saturated Fat Ratio	Unsaturated Fat to Saturated Fat Ratio
2.5:1 O-6 to O-3 ratio	11:1 O-6 to O-3 ratio
Dietary Cholesterol Intake	Dietary Cholesterol Intake
480 mg/day	480 mg/day
Serum (Blood) Cholesterol	Serum (Blood) Cholesterol
125 mg/dL	250mg/dL

SAD (STANDARD AMERICAN DIET)

SAD refers to the Standard American Diet. And it is nothing short of sad. If you were to do a quantitative analysis of the standard American diet, the macronutrient ratio would average 45-50% carbohydrate, 40-45% fat, and 10-15% protein. That doesn't tell you a lot, except the fat is too high and the protein too low. It doesn't describe why the SAD diet is a disaster. But if you were to move from a quantitative analysis to a qualitative analysis, your eyes would open to exactly how poorly Americans really eat.

The USDA reports that the top nine foods eaten by Americans are: whole cow's milk, 2% milk, processed American cheese, white bread, white flour, white rolls, refined sugar, colas, and ground (corn-fed) beef. None of these so-called foods were eaten by our Paleolithic ancestors, but they all contribute to our current obese and diseased state.

If you were to do a qualitative analysis of SAD, you'd find that typical Americans eat far too many refined carbohydrates, not enough fiber, vitamins, minerals, antioxidants, or phytochemicals (healthy chemical compounds, such as beta-carotene, that occur naturally in plants), too many low-quality fats and trans fats, not enough healthy omega-3 fats, too many chemical residues, and not enough nutrients overall.

Here's a look at a typical day's nutrition for a twenty-first century high school athlete—this might seem familiar to you:

You wake up around 7 a.m. still tired and you're rushing to get to school on time. You skip breakfast and it's not until lunch that you scarf down your first meal—either fast food or greasy, processed cafeteria food (like pizza or chicken nuggets). You wash it down with a carton of milk or a soda. After school, you slam down an energy drink, a soda, or an expensive coffee drink to help you make it through the rest of your day. When you get home at night, you sit down with your family for a home-cooked dinner of either some sort of animal protein like chicken or ground beef, a starch like pasta or pizza, juice, and a dessert like pie or a bowl of ice cream. You then stay up until midnight or later watching TV, playing on the Internet, or playing video games, only to repeat the same process the next day. Sound familiar?

Most of these foods weren't even in existence during Paleolithic times. Now, I am not saying you need to drop all of your favorite foods and desserts completely, but you need to redefine what you consider your staple foods and consider the others an occasional snack or treat. You can still enjoy being a teenager, but if you truly understood how much your nutritional choices were affecting your performance both in sports and in the classroom, let alone your overall happiness, you'd be motivated to make this transformation.

Key takeaways from this chapter:

- Nutritional quality (the source of the food you eat) is way more important than nutritional quantity (the calorie count and macronutrient percentages: grams of protein, carbohydrate and fat) of the foods you eat.
- Nature made it easy for us to know what to eat. Our access to food and on-the-go lifestyle demands have messed it up.
- Paleolithic nutrition basically consists of consuming lean meats and fish (from animals that eat what they are supposed to), seasonal vegetables, small amounts of fruits, nuts and seeds, and healthy oils.
- You don't need to drop all of your favorite foods and desserts completely, but you need to redefine what you consider your

staple foods and consider the others an occasional snack or treat.

Chapter 4

Chickens Don't Have Nuggets—Roosters Do!
The problems with processed foods, and why if it doesn't spoil quickly,
you shouldn't eat it!

Why is it acceptable to feed our youth things we wouldn't consider adult food? I've never sat down at a business dinner and been served chicken nuggets, macaroni and cheese, or a peanut butter and jelly sandwich and a juice box. This paradox is the foundation of the second secret a champion knows: chickens don't have nuggets... roosters do!

It seems like a basic concept, but when it comes to healthy nutrition, it is actually revolutionary. Americans have a strong disassociation from where our food originates. We cut chicken up into cute, single-bite servings, bread it, deep-fry it, and call it a nugget. Besides chicken nuggets, there are other major problems we have with modern-day processed, convenient foods. In a 2007 study, 61% of competitive foods (foods sold outside of the School Meals program, including in vending machines, a la carte items, school store/canteen items, etc.) offered in high schools were fried and high in fat. These calorie-dense, nutrition-poor foods accounted for 83% of all food sold. [5] Also, traditional school lunches and convenient foods have too many chemical residues. For example, while sliced turkey meat from an organic turkey may be healthy for you, typical deli lunch meat contains up to 600 different chemicals, is high in salt, nitrates, nitrites, preservatives, artificial colors and flavors, and anabolic hormones they feed animals. Moreover, classifications of what is a fruit and what is a vegetable are way off base. **For example, French fries are the most common vegetable consumed by children and make up one-fourth of children's vegetable intake.** Juice, which typically lacks important fiber found in whole fruits, accounts for 40% of children's daily fruit intake. [6]

Even counting French fries and juice as vegetable and fruit sources, most children and teens are not eating enough fruits and vegetables. Fewer than one in ten high school students get the recommended amounts of fruits and vegetables daily. Another major problem with packaged, processed, convenient foods is the high sodium levels required for these products to have a long shelf life. Most Americans consume more than double the amount of the daily recommended intake of sodium (salt). The majority of sodium we consume comes from salt added to the food supply (not from salt we add at the table).

The major requirements for a healthy school lunch option that works for parents and kids alike is that it must be delicious, healthy, convenient, and economical. Rather than feeling like you need to change everything you do today, start by implementing a few foundational principles:

1. If it doesn't spoil quickly, you shouldn't eat it! All Paleolithic foods, from lean animal protein to vegetables and fruits to healthy oils, were all once living food.
2. Follow the universal rule of proper animal nutrition, which is to eat only the food that nature intended you to eat in the portions

you would come across in nature. For example, in nature, pre-Agricultural Revolution, you would not come across a peanut butter and jelly sandwich. You would, however, come across almonds. In their natural form, almonds have protective shells on them. It would take you a long time to de-shell almonds, and maybe you could eat twelve of them in half an hour. However, these days you can go to nearly any grocery store, grab a large bag full of de-shelled almonds, and eat thirty of them in under two minutes.

3. Follow the unprocessed principle, which is the only universal principal across all major dietary systems. The unprocessed principle states that you should eat as close to original source of food as possible.

Below is an example of processing:

- Organic fruit —> non-organic fruit —> fresh juice —> filtered/pasteurized juice —> filtered/pasteurized juice with colors, flavors, sugar
- Organic whole grain —> non-organic whole grain —> whole grain flour product (i.e. whole wheat bread or pasta) —> refined flour product (i.e. white bread or pasta) —> refined flour (i.e. cakes, cookies, etc.)
- If you eat grains, the unprocessed principal would move you toward an organic whole grain. More processed leads to exposure of grain to oxygen, which leads to rancid lipids (fats). Moreover, you have no idea how long

bread was sitting on the shelf, nor how long the flour was sitting in the bakery, nor how it was stored or heated.

4. Avoid artificial sweeteners.

    What's wrong with artificial sweeteners? According to Dr. Joseph Mercola, "They've been approved by the FDA, they are on nearly every table in every restaurant nationwide, and they're in nearly every low-calorie soda, snack food, or dessert food on the market..."

    - They are completely unnatural
    - There is no long-term data showing the safety of artificial sweeteners
    - Unnecessary to the diet
    - Illegal in many countries
    - Have a long history of causing health problems

There are healthy, great-tasting alternatives". [7] Healthy alternatives include raw honey, agave, Stevia, Xylitol, Erythritol and Luo Han Guo fruit extract (also know as Monk fruit).

HOW TO EAT OUT HEALTHILY FOR YOUR ON-THE-GO LIFESTYLE

People are eating out more than ever before. When people eat out, they consume more calories and processed foods and fewer fruits and vegetables than when they prepare meals at home. On any given day, one in every three children eats a fast-food meal, according to a new U.S. study. Children who eat fast food consume, on average, an additional 187 calories daily, researchers found. While that may not sound like much—it's the equivalent of a medium soft drink—it translates into an additional six pounds a year in excess body weight and goes a long way toward explaining the skyrocketing rates of childhood obesity. Dr. Ludwig (director of the obesity program at Children's Hospital Boston, and lead author of a study on the dietary habits of children published in the journal *Pediatrics*) said children who routinely eat fast-food meals consume not only more calories, but also more fat (including trans fats), more sugar, and more salt; they also eat fewer vegetables, consume less fiber and drink less milk.

Dr. Ludwig noted that in 1970, fast food accounted for less than 2% of the caloric intake (or energy) of children; by the early 1990s, it accounted for more than 10%; new research shows that, today, children are getting up to 38% of their energy from burgers, fries and other fatty foods. He pointed out an earlier study that showed that children who eat fast food more than twice a week are 86% more likely to end up obese than those who rarely or never consume fast food.

So how do you handle eating out healthily while still accommodating your on-the-go-lifestyle? It's actually quite easy. First, you need to realize that the best fast food restaurant is actually the health food store. You can run into nearly any health food store and order either a hot meal of some sort of animal protein, like chicken, turkey, beef, or fish, or some cooked vegetables, and pick up a piece of fruit on your way to check out. Alternatively, you can easily make a salad with chicken, tuna, or eggs at the salad bar. Lastly, you can walk up to the deli counter and order a few ounces of organic sliced turkey or beef with a piece of fruit. All of these options are just as fast and convenient as a drive-thru and are much healthier.

But what about when you go out to a sit-down restaurant? What are the best tips to stick to your game plan when you're out of your comfort zone?

1. **Snack Before You Go.** Have a handful of trail mix or an apple with peanut butter at home before you leave for dinner. Typically, an hour passes from the time you leave for the restaurant to the time you're seated and your food arrives at your table.

2. **Don't Carb-Load Before Your Entrée Arrives.** Have the waiter remove bread or chips and order a salad appetizer with an oil-based dressing, as the high fiber and fat content will keep you from overindulging. Start chugging the water as soon as you sit down to curb your appetite.

3. **Base Your Meal Around Lean Protein.** Find an entrée that is protein-packed, with chicken, fish, turkey, or lean steak, rather than noodle or bread-based. This protein will provide you with sustained energy, as well as serve as the building blocks to repair or replace every cell in your body.

4. **Substitute Veggies for Grains.** Side dishes tend to be larger in size than the entrees they accompany. Instead of going for the French fries, rice, or mashed potatoes, choose cooked veggies like broccoli, grilled asparagus, portabella mushrooms or spinach.

5. **Dietary Fat Will Leave You Satisfied.** One of the biggest
    mistakes in the English language is using the word fat for both
    dietary fat and body fat. Excess glycogen from grains and sugary
    foods are stored as body fat, unlike the small quantities of
    healthy dietary fats. Most "healthy" restaurant meals leave you
    unsatisfied, as they lack healthy fats. Rather than reaching for
    grain products (bread, rice, tortillas, etc.) that will simply leave
    you bloated, add some avocado, healthy oils, or nuts and seeds to
    your salad or cooked vegetables; they will leave you satisfied.

6. **Don't Feel Obligated To Lick Your Plate Clean.** It has been
    engrained in our brains since childhood to finish all the food on
    our plates. As children, we're guilted with "Don't waste food—
    there are starving people in Africa (or Asia)." While intentions
    are good, restaurant portions in this country are out-of-control
    big. In Africa, they must be telling their children, "Don't
    overeat—there are obese people in America!" If the portions are
    too big, share or bring a doggie bag home.

THE HOUR TO DEVOUR

I completely appreciate that you're still a kid and you enjoy your
"cheat" foods like pizza, pasta, candy, and ice cream. There is nothing
wrong with occasionally eating these foods. The quickest way to get
someone to eat more junk food is to completely restrict it. The key is
to plan your indulgences as best as possible and eat real food for
your staple meals. This can be achieved by incorporating an hour to
devour into your lifestyle.

Hour to Devour™: Once or maybe twice a week, when you "go to town" and eat ANYTHING you've been craving that doesn't move (and isn't poisonous/toxic... although in actuality, they are :). This can include ice cream, pizza, pasta, candy, fast food or other bread products. The hour when you look at the menu and say, "Yes, please!"*

*Warning: Overindulgence usually leads to initial joy followed by regret in the form of upset stomach, lethargy, gas, bloating, and a multitude of other temporary symptoms that just "aren't fun." The Hour to Devour™ is not included in the program of diabetics, gastric bypass clients, heart patients, anyone with severe food allergies, celiac disease, or anyone with an exceptionally weak immune system. Make sure you consult a physician before incorporating an Hour to Devour into your eating plan.

Why incorporate The Hour to Devour™ into your healthy lifestyle?

- It eliminates the diet mentality
- It keeps you "human"
- It helps set weekly objectives
- It prevents you from "falling off the health wagon"
- It improves awareness of how different foods affect your body

The Hour to Devour™ can remain part of your program even after you have achieved your goals. Most people start out overindulging during their hour but quickly learn that all they need is a small indulgence—like a piece of pizza or a small ice cream cone—to keep them from feeling deprived of their favorite foods and committed to a healthy lifestyle.

Key takeaways from this chapter:

- It should be unacceptable to feed our youth things we wouldn't consider adult food.
- Fewer than one in ten high school students get the recommended amounts of fruits and vegetables daily.
- If it doesn't spoil quickly, don't eat it!
- Simply follow the universal rule of proper animal nutrition, which is to eat only the food that nature intended you to eat in the portions you would come across in nature.
- Follow the unprocessed principle, which states that you should eat as close to original source of food as possible.
- The key is to plan your indulgences as best as possible and eat real food for your staple meals. This can be achieved by incorporating an Hour to Devour into your lifestyle.

Chapter 5

How Much Does a Zebra Weigh?

Why you should throw out your scale, stop measuring your food, and transform the way you view your cuisine

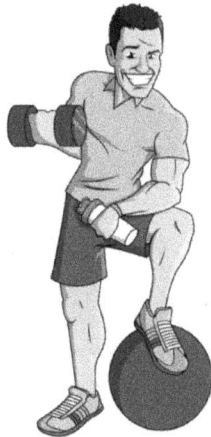

"Me, Coach Kyle"

One of the biggest secrets to understanding real nutrition is to recognize that we as humans are part of the animal kingdom. If you look at the basics of zoology, you'll see that the rest of the animal kingdom has it right—then you'll laugh at what most people put on their plates.

Although humans are one of the most intelligent, resourceful and thriving animals on the planet, we are also the sickest, most overstressed and unintentionally fat animals on the planet. While there are a few other animals with high body fat, nature designed these animals to store excess body fat as fuel and to keep them warm in the harsh conditions of their environment. For example, whales are mammals just like humans and have a body temperature similar to ours. To adapt to water as cold as 29° Fahrenheit, they have a layer of fat under their skin called blubber which they use as fuel and which keeps them insulated. Bears also store excess body fat for reserve energy and to keep them warm as they hibernate for months during the long, cold winter.

Since humans have become the only unintentionally fat animal in the animal kingdom, let's examine animals that are healthy, fit and conditioned to uncover their secrets.

I'd like to introduce you to my friend, Champ the Chimp. Champ will be your guide to unlocking the health and fitness secrets of the animal kingdom. Why is Champ qualified to talk to you about fitness and nutrition? Chimpanzees are hunter-gatherer omnivores (meaning that chimps eat a diet of both plant and animal sources) just like us. Chimps also share 94% of our biophysical characteristics. You won't find an obese chimp in nature. Chimps are also fitness gurus, as they are on average roughly five to seven times stronger than humans, display effortless agility and balance, and do not suffer from the same diet and lifestyle-related diseases as we do. Chimps eat a diet that is very similar to the way our Paleolithic (ancient) ancestors used to eat before modern societies began farming and processing, giving rise to the eating patterns that led to today's health problems. The main difference is that chimpanzees don't have access to all of the delicious animal protein sources that we do, so they have to hunt insects for their main protein source. Without further ado, I give you Champ the Chimp.

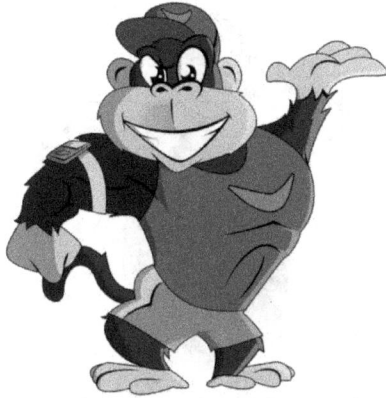

"Champ The Chimp"

CHAMP:

Hi! I've met many humans who treat me like family when they visit my home in the rainforest in Africa. Yet other bad humans hunt us and are making us lose our habitat. While I'm still here on this planet, I want to let you good people in on a little secret: how you can effortlessly lose weight and gain boundless energy by going back to your roots.

It's been hard watching humans losing the battle of the bulge. Especially, it's been so hard watching innocent children fall victim to the obesity crisis. I just had to get involved. And since having my little girl, Chi, I realize that proper education and healthy habits must start in early childhood before the commercial food industry gets their hands on you, leaving you confused, frustrated and desperate.

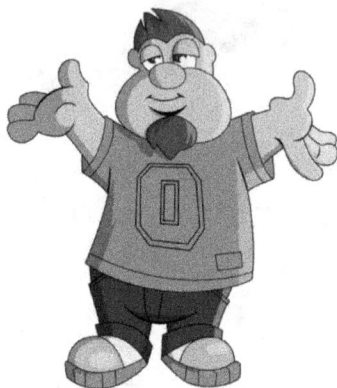

"SAD (Struggling American Dieter)"

For instance, meet my friend, SAD. His name stands for Struggling American Dieter. SAD is a stress case. He works way too many hours and never seems to get enough sleep. SAD is constantly on some new fad diet. On one hand, he thinks he knows everything about eating and exercise since he has succeeded in losing weight in the past many times over (only to gain it all back). SAD watches a lot of fitness TV shows, reads a lot of fitness magazines, and believes that weight loss is easy and that it's all about keeping your calorie intake lower than the calories you use each day. On the other hand, SAD's weight always comes back on, and then some! SAD goes through bouts of being really dedicated to his eating and workouts and then completely giving up and falling off the wagon. Like most of you out there, SAD was frustrated with all of the conflicting information on healthy eating and fitness and was about ready to give up—before he met me.

Let's face it: SAD is not alone. Most people have a little bit of SAD in them. Obesity is an epidemic, and the chances that you're going succeed in staying healthy with a fad diet are slim to none. Remember, the first the letters in diet are D-I-E!

You may be thinking, "I'm still a kid," or, "I'm not fat. Why do I need to learn how to eat healthy now?" It's because habits are formed when you're young. And if you start applying these secrets to your life, your goals will change from losing weight to creating habits that will help you live a healthy lifestyle.

Humans need to understand that skinny doesn't always mean healthy. Just like overweight kids, many skinny kids are weak, uncoordinated, unhealthy, and are loaded up on so much sugar that they're unable to pay attention in school. Weight by itself is not a good health indicator. The goal is for you to be healthy, happy and strong—just like my daughter, Chi.

So imagine you're on safari in my home continent of Africa. You're alert and your eyes are wide open to observing animals in their natural state. First, let's look at the herbivores. Pretend for a moment you were somehow able to line up 1,000 zebras side by side and compare their physical traits. What would you notice first?

Well, they're all fairly similar looking, although their most famous feature, their stripes, come in different patterns unique to each individual zebra and serve as a sort of protective coloration, making it difficult to distinguish the zebra against certain backgrounds and hard to determine where one zebra ends and another begins. Most zebras are about the same height (between 3.5 and 5 feet tall measured from the ground to the top of the shoulder, with females being typically shorter than males, similar to humans.) [8]

You'll also notice that they're all lean, fit, conditioned animals in their natural state. While some may have more muscle mass or slightly larger bone structure, and others may be thinner because they haven't had access to enough food, you'll not find an obese zebra in nature. I'll say that once again, just to let it soak in: you will not find an obese zebra in nature. Why is this? How come these animals, without any of the resources you humans have access to, don't have the obesity issues or the mass disease issues that humans have? Well, let's analyze them a little further.

Check out my gorgeous friend, Zoe the Zebra. Zoe is a beautiful, fit, high-energy and fearless creature, yet she's still graceful—if Beyoncé were a zebra, she'd be Zoe.

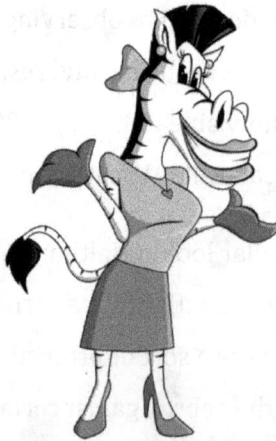

"Zoe The Zebra"

SAD:

So how much does a zebra weigh?

CHAMP:

SAD, you know it's not polite to ask a girl her weight. Fortunately, zebras don't care. According to Zoe the Zebra, the answer is "Who cares?!" Technically, a female zebra weighs between 440 and 600 pounds, with males averaging from 700 to 990 pounds. [9] Yet, there is a more meaningful answer to the question "How much does a zebra weigh?" Zoe and her fellow zebras don't know what a scale is, nor do they care. If a zebra came across a scale in the wilderness, they might smell it to see if it was edible—but after that, a scale is useless to a zebra. It doesn't dictate whether or not Zoe the Zebra is healthy, happy, in good physical condition or physically attractive. Nor should humans think it indicates these things!

Now, I'm not saying there's anything wrong with taking pride in your appearance. However, scale weight has nothing to do with attractiveness, and no other animal knows or cares about its weight. Zoe the Zebra won't pick her mate based on how much he weighs. Likewise, if you kids walk down the hall in school or see a cute boy or girl at the mall or the gym, you wouldn't know or care what he or she weighs. You wouldn't think, "That cute boy is 182 pounds," or, "That pretty girl must be 131 pounds." In reality, you'd just make a judgment of "attractive" or "not attractive." Ideas of attractiveness have nothing to do with scale weight, but are more about how someone takes care of themselves, their style, their confidence and how they carry themselves, and genetic features like hair and eye color that we have no control over. Nor does Zoe the Zebra have a better quality of life or better health because she weighs 472 pounds instead of 511 pounds. Yet for some reason, you humans obsess about your scale weight, and have been led to believe that a number on a scale can measure happiness.

Can you relate to this scenario? It's 7:00 A.M. You've been on a diet for a whole week and have been exercising like crazy. You walk into the bathroom and step onto this magical box that you call a scale and think to yourself, "Oh please, magic box, show me a number lower than the number I saw yesterday so that I'll know that I've lost weight and am therefore more attractive, more successful, more loved, and happier." Many of the most popular reality television shows glamorize this magical scale as a sort of Wizard of Oz that will make us successful in life if we can just hit the right number. Come on, does this make any sense? Yet many Americans obsess about their scale weight and let it dictate their happiness. Weight loss should be a by-product of living a healthy lifestyle, not the end goal.

So let's get back to Zoe the Zebra, because understanding how ridiculous scale weight is as a measure for health, success, or happiness is just the tip of the iceberg.

SAD:

What does Zoe the Zebra eat?

CHAMP:

Zoe is an herbivore, meaning she eats only plant life. Specifically, she eats wild grasses—but as adaptable grazers, zebras can also eat shrubs, herbs, twigs, leaves and bark during times of scarcity. These wild grasses are made up of quality protein, fiber, and healthy oils to keep Zoe properly nourished and energized.

Zoe the Zebra has a matched set of incisors and mobile lips that grip a tuft of grass while her front teeth cut it off. Her back teeth (molars) grind the grass. Zoe's digestive system has intestines that twist and turn even more than humans' do. Zebras graze all day long in order to get enough nutrition. Like humans, zebras are very social animals and they travel in herds, so Zoe learned what to eat from observing the other members of her herd family.

SAD:

How many calories does Zoe the Zebra eat?

CHAMP:

Who cares?! As you just learned in the chapter "Stop Counting Calories—It's Making You Fat And Weak," humans are the only animals of whom the majority is consistently sick and fat, and yet humans are the only animals who count calories. No other animal has any idea what a calorie is.

SAD:

How much does Zoe the Zebra eat?

CHAMP:

Zoe consumes approximately 20 pounds of food per day, primarily in the form of grass. To eat this much food, Zoe the Zebra spends 60 to 80% of her day grazing in grasslands. [9]

Zoe can eat all this grass yet remain fit and conditioned because the calorie content of the foods she eats is very low yet nutrient-dense, high in vitamins, minerals, and fiber. Same with the calorie content of the type of foods humans and chimps were meant to eat.

SAD:

When does Zoe the Zebra eat?

CHAMP:

A zebra eats when it's hungry, of course. Yet the answer isn't so simple for humans. Humans eat for a variety of reasons far beyond simply being hungry. You eat when you're hungry, but you also tend to eat for emotional reasons, like when you're depressed, stressed, having cravings, are "hormonal," when you're celebrating, bored, lonely and need to be comforted, when you're trying to put on muscle, in a social setting, and when it's "the polite thing to do."

SAD:

When does Zoe the Zebra stop eating?

CHAMP:

Zebras stop eating when they're full and satisfied. Humans, on the other hand, tend to eat until they're stuffed and bloated, and they can't recognize the difference. When you get to reading later in this book about what starch versus fiber and dietary fat do in the body, you'll understand the difference.

SAD:

What time of day does Zoe the Zebra eat?

CHAMP:

Zoe doesn't know or care about time. She's too busy living in the moment. Zebras are grazers, which means they eat continuously throughout the day, depleting the food supply in one area before moving on to the next area. No other animal besides humans keeps track of time or sets a time of day to stop eating. I have yet to see Zoe step away from a healthy, luscious green pasture and inform her heard to stop eating, as it's already 8 p.m. This is why people should not watch the clock or try to eat only before a certain time. Each person is an individual and has different times when they need to wake up and go to bed, based on numerous factors like career, family, deadlines for projects, and social obligations. If you're not feeding yourself when you're awake, your body will store body fat for future use, since it doesn't know when it's going to be fed again. This is called going into starvation mode. Your metabolism is like a bonfire; if you constantly add kindling to the fire (i.e. eat small, frequent meals) your metabolism will become stronger, hotter, and more powerful. Simply eat more of the right foods when you're awake and hungry and listen to your body.

Zoe the Zebra likes to keep it simple and follows the universal rule of proper animal nutrition, which is to eat only the food that nature intend you to eat in the portions you come across in nature.

SAD:

I bet Zoe the Zebra is lean because she's always on her feet and runs around playing all day long. If zebras had to work all day long, like me, they'd be fat.

CHAMP:

Well, here's another example from nature that will prove that statement wrong. Let's take a look at the carnivores now, using lions as an example. Meet my friend, Lex the Lion. Just like Zoe and her fellow zebras, you'll not find a fat lion in nature. Some may be bigger, with more muscle mass or bigger bone structure, while others may be smaller and malnourished due to scarcity; but in nature, lions are high in explosive energy for when they hunt food or defend their pride, and are fit and conditioned just like zebras. Lex is built like a brick house, yet he's more agile and explosive than an NFL linebacker.

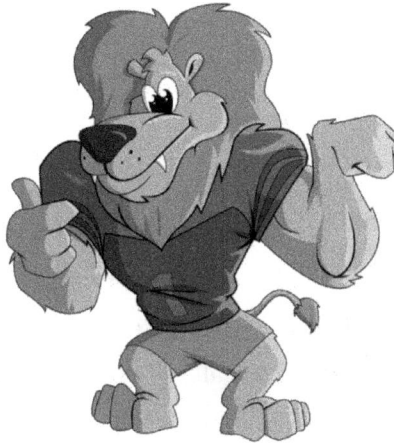

"Lex The Lion"

SAD:

How much does Lex the Lion exercise in a typical day? He's got all that muscle and no body fat. I bet he spends the entire day working out!

CHAMP:

Not at all. Lex is a typical male lion. He sleeps up to 80% of the day, while his wife Lucy does the hunting and raises the kids. But he still makes time to exercise. Lions spend an average of two hours a day walking and 50 minutes eating. [10]

SAD:

So how much does Lex the Lion weigh?

CHAMP:

You know the answer. It's "Who cares?!"

SAD:

How many calories does Lex the Lion eat?

CHAMP: Again, who cares?! A much more important question is, what does Lex the Lion eat? Zebras! But don't worry, he and Zoe are friends. While he feels terrible about eating zebras like Zoe, Lex is at peace with it, as he knows it's the way nature designed him. Besides zebras, lions eat other wild animals, all of which eat what they're supposed to eat. This is the whole basis of the food chain. Animals at the top of the food chain are supposed to eat animals on the next step of the food chain, which eat whatever they are designed by nature to eat. You'll learn more about this in the chapter "The Manipulated Food Chain: You Are What You Eat."

Lex's digestive track is short and simple like a pipe, as he eats and chews meat then eliminates most of the fat right away. Zebras have flat teeth that are good for tearing up leaves, but Lex the Lion has sharp teeth that are able to rip apart flesh. You humans have both molars like Zoe the Zebra and canine teeth like Lex the Lion.

SAD:

So when does Lex the Lion eat?

CHAMP:

Whenever he can get a good kill and pass the meat on to his family.

All of the above questions have common sense answers, just like for zebras. Yet when it comes to human nutrition, common sense is thrown out the window and replaced with fad diets and trends that make no sense when you look at the natural way of things.

You humans are a combination of the lions and zebras. Although many people feel superior to animals, nutritionally speaking you're part of the animal kingdom: hunter-gatherer omnivores who eat for strength, speed, and endurance just like us chimpanzees!

Chapter 6

Breakfast Is the Most Important Meal of the Day
Small, protein-packed meals kick-start your metabolism

So, what did you have for breakfast this morning? A bagel and cream cheese? Cereal? Nothing? It's true that breakfast is the most important meal of the day. Multiple studies have demonstrated that when teens skip breakfast, the nutritional quality of their diets decreases and they actually gain body fat. Eating breakfast keeps your energy levels high throughout the day, increasing your mental focus, and your reaction time. Breakfast is another perfect example of how nutritional quality is more important than nutritional quantity.

So many Americans think that if they skip breakfast, they will consume fewer calories over the course of the day, and that in turn will help them lose weight. Yet research consistently proves otherwise. By not eating breakfast, you are robbing your body of the most important meal of the day. When you skip breakfast, your body goes into starvation mode and holds onto stubborn body fat, because it doesn't know when it's getting its next meal. Remember, your metabolism is like a bonfire. If you put all of your wood on the bonfire at once, it will quickly burn out. You need to start off with a solid foundation and add a moderate amount of fuel to the fire every few hours. When it comes to your internal bonfire, breakfast is the foundation. The trick is to eat small meals every three to four hours. If you starve yourself and then eat too much at one time, you'll feel stuffed, bloated and lethargic, and your body will hold onto that excess fuel as body fat.

Teens who skip breakfast have a significantly higher risk of obesity. According to research published in the journal *Pediatrics*, teens who skipped breakfast were five pounds heavier on average, ate less healthily during the day, and exercised less frequently than those who ate breakfast. [11] Moreover, according to the American Journal of Epidemiology, people who regularly skipped breakfast had 4.5 times the risk of obesity as those who regularly consumed breakfast. On the other hand, people who eat more often throughout the day typically have a lower obesity risk. [12]

What's even more important than eating breakfast? What you eat when you eat breakfast. Most breakfast options are outrageously bad for you. Typical breakfast options consist of low-nutrient garbage including pancakes, waffles, sugar cereal, bagels, muffins, toast and doughnuts, with sides like bacon, sausage and juice. In many cases, I'd rather see you eat ice cream for breakfast—at least you'd be getting quality protein and decent dietary fat, rather than simply sugar, starch and low-quality fat. Not that ice cream is a healthy option or a good choice, but most breakfast cereals are worse.

For example, sugary cereals targeted to youth are loaded with refined carbohydrates and sugar. According to a March 2010 article in *USA Today*, most cereals for children contain as much as 65% more sugar than adult cereals. A 2009 analysis by Consumer Reports found that eleven popular breakfast cereals contain at least 40% sugar. That's as much sugar as you'd get in a glazed doughnut! This report also notes that many sugary cereals are marketed heavily to children—and that many children tend to pour more cereal for themselves than the suggested serving size. That means that many of the kids and teens who aren't sleeping through breakfast are eating brightly colored refined white flour and sugar for breakfast before they head off to school each day.

Since it's not practical to hunt down a buffalo and throw it on the barbeque at 7 a.m. before class, what are the alternatives? How can you make breakfast if you're always in a rush in the morning? And who wants to eat meat in the morning? Try a delicious, convenient, natural, grass-fed whey protein-based meal replacement shake. Grass-fed whey comes from cows that are 100% pasture-raised and are not fed hormones or antibiotics. Just make sure your shake is a complete meal, like FIT 365®, with healthy fibers, oils, enzymes and no artificial ingredients, rather than just a protein shake. Remember, all meals should consist of healthy proteins, fiber, and dietary fat.

Make an omelet when you have extra time in the morning. A study in the International Journal of Obesity showed that eating two eggs for breakfast as part of a reduced-calorie diet helps overweight people lose more weight and feel more energetic than eating a bagel of equal calories for breakfast. [13] This study supports previous research that showed people who ate eggs for breakfast felt more satisfied and ate fewer calories at the following meal. Compared to the subjects who ate a bagel for breakfast with an equal number of calories, men and women who consumed two eggs for breakfast as part of a reduced-calorie diet lost 65%more weight, exhibited a 61% greater reduction in BMI, and reported higher energy levels. [14]

Key takeaways from this chapter:

- Multiple studies have demonstrated that when teens skip breakfast, the nutritional quality of their diets decreases and they actually gain body fat.
- Eating breakfast keeps your energy levels high throughout the day, increasing your mental focus and your reaction time.
- Try a delicious, convenient, natural, grass-fed whey protein-based meal replacement shake like FIT 365® for breakfast, or make an omelet when you have the time.

Chapter 7

What Protein, Carbs, and Fat Do in the Body

End the guesswork on what it takes to make a complete meal

At some point in the history of American diets, all three macronutrients—protein, carbohydrates, and fats—have been demonized as being bad for you. If you were to listen to everything you hear from every side, you would be left eating cardboard! Most teens think they know what protein, carbohydrates, and fats are and what they do in their bodies—as do most adults. Yet the truth is, both groups are far off the mark.

	What We Think	The Truth
Protein	Gives you muscles	Sustained energy
		Muscle building and sparing
		Building blocks of every cell in your body
		It's what you absorb that counts
		You are what you eat
Sugar	Gives you energy	Energy spikes then

		crashes
		Stored in fat cells
		Not the ideal fuel source
		An addictive drug
Fiber	Makes you regular	Promotes healthy bowel movements
		Keeps you from overeating
		Leaves you full
Starch	Required for energy	Turns into sugar rapidly in the body
	Makes a complete meal	Adequate amounts found in certain veggies
	Leaves you full and satisfied	Most high-starch foods make you fat
Fat	Makes you fat	Satiates you
		Body's preferred energy source
		Helps burn body fat

PROTEIN

Most people think that eating protein builds muscles. In reality, that's only a small part of the benefits of protein. Protein breaks down into essential amino acids—which your body requires but cannot create—and non-essential amino acids. These amino acids build and repair every cell in your body. Protein is responsible not only for muscle building but for muscle sparing. When you're in a caloric deficit and trying to lose body fat, you need to constantly eat protein so you're not losing muscle while you're losing fat. This way your body will utilize your fat stores for energy instead of your muscle. Remember, your goals should never focus on weight loss; they should focus on fat loss.

Not all protein sources are the same. There's a big difference between how many grams of protein you digest and how many you actually absorb. Here are a few key points when it comes to protein sources:

1. Whey, egg, dairy, and animal meats (in that order) have the highest bio-availability (are the highest absorbed and best utilized) as protein sources. Vegetable proteins (nuts, veggies, and beans) have the lowest.
2. Avoid all non-fermented soy products at all times (nearly all soy protein products, except miso, tempeh, natto and tamari).
3. You don't need to avoid red meat as long as it's lean and ideally grass-fed (from cows that only eat grass). Red meat is a good source of iron and zinc—minerals which many people

are lacking. Healthy lean red meats include flank steak, top sirloin, filet mignon, extra lean hamburger (no more than 7% fat), London broil, and chuck steak, as well as game animals such as ostrich and bison.

4. If you choose to avoid animal meat, use whey or egg white protein powder, cheese and eggs to meet your protein needs.

CARBOHYDRATES

Carbohydrates include fruits, vegetables, grains, breads and cereals. Yet the carbohydrates nature truly intended for human consumption are vegetables, primarily, and fruit secondarily. The grain industry has done a fantastic job convincing Americans that grains, breads, and cereals are the only carbohydrates. In truth, 30% to 60% of your carbohydrates can easily come from vegetables and fruits. Glycogen management is the key to successful weight management. Therefore, carbohydrate intake must be monitored and kept in moderation. Carbohydrates are important, as they provide vitamins, minerals, fiber, and energy to fuel your body. It's important to maintain a balance between acid and alkaline foods. Acid/alkaline balance is one of the key indicators of optimal health. Fruits and vegetables are nature's main sources of alkaline foods.

Carbohydrate energy is like a roller coaster; it shoots you straight to the top, but drops you right back down. It's not a good source of energy. Sugar, fiber, starch, and micronutrients are the four subcategories of carbs. Micronutrients are the vitamins, minerals, antioxidants, phytochemicals (plant-based nutrients), and all of the other things we haven't even discovered yet. All of these are found in vegetables and fruits.

SUGAR

Most people think that sugar is the body's preferred source of energy. This is far from the truth for the majority of people. Most bodies run best on healthy oils and protein. As mentioned earlier, sugar spikes your energy then lets you crash. This is a sign of poor sugar utilization. When sugar enters the body, it's broken down into glycogen. Your liver utilizes some of the glycogen and some is stored in your muscle cells. It then runs through your bloodstream to be used for your daily activities, such as living and exercise. Muscle cells are small and finite in size. However, fat cells can be infinite in size, so the leftover glycogen is stored in your fat cells. Why won't the glycogen just leave your system? Because your body looks at fat cells and sugar this way: once sugar enters your body, it wants to hold onto it for an emergency—in case you get chased or cannot eat. Your body doesn't realize that it doesn't need to hold onto the fat.

Sugar is addictive—it can be just as addictive as nearly any drug. In truth, sugar is a drug—it's a quick-fix drug. Once you have it, you want more, and if you have too much you feel sick. It's one of those drugs that you will start craving after every meal and throughout the day. Just go cold turkey for a few days and the cravings will stop.

FIBER

We're all well aware that fiber makes you regular. I know, it's kind of funny, so you can laugh now. Yes, fiber promotes healthy bowel movements. But more importantly, fiber is nature's safety mechanism to keep you from overeating. It leaves you feeling full. For example, how come grass-fed cows are skinny while corn and soy-fed cows are obese? Because unlike grains and soy, grass is loaded with tons of fiber, so inactive cows can remain lean and conditioned even without exercise! Yet grain products take all of the credit for being high in fiber. This is not the case in comparison with vegetables or fruits. For example, if I were to give you $1,000 to eat six servings of white rice (each serving being the size of a golf ball), at 80 calories per serving you'd be ingesting 480 calories and only 3.6 grams of fiber. And I bet you could probably eat double that for an additional $1,000. However, if I were to give you $1,000 to eat six apples, it'd be next to impossible because apples are so fiber-rich. But if you did manage to eat them all, you'd have consumed 19.8 grams of fiber and only 360 calories. What noise does an apple make when you consume it? Crunch crunch! That's the fiber talking to you. This is why veggie-eating herbivores are thin in nature. Fruits and vegetables have almost four times the fiber and less than one-third the calories of most grains!

STARCH

Starch is the one component that usually leaves the average American clueless. Most Americans believe a high-starch side dish is required for energy and leaves you full and satisfied. This is a marketing fallacy and the furthest thing from the truth. The truth is that fiber leaves you full and most starch leaves you bloated and wanting more.

But what is starch? Starch is the hidden carbohydrate that can make you obese if eaten in excess. It's primarily found in seeds, fruits, tubers, roots and the stem pith of plants—notably in corn, potatoes, wheat, and rice. While there are certain high-starch vegetables, including yams, sweet potatoes, and squash, for the sake of distinction I'm referring to the starch in grain products like bread, pasta and other processed complex carbs.

Starch rapidly turns into sugar in the body. This is where a lot of people mess up on their nutrition programs. They read a nutrition label with only 2g of sugar and think the product is low in sugar. Then they see 5g of fiber and think the product is high in fiber. But in actuality, the product has a total of 35g of carbs. If you subtract the 5g of fiber and the 2g of sugar from the 35g of total carbs, you're left with 28g of carbs. What are these other 28g? They're starch! All starchy foods are glycemic foods, meaning they rapidly turn into sugar in your body. So if you take the 2g of sugar and add it to the 28g of starch, you've now consumed 30g of carbs, which your body will convert into sugar. And most of this sugar and starch will end up in your fat cells as stored energy.

You'll learn more about the dangers of starch in the chapter called "Ask Any Farmer: Grains, Sugar, and Soy Make You Sick and Overweight!"

FAT

One of the biggest mistakes in the English language is the use of the word fat to describe both body fat and dietary fat. Most of us have been raised to believe that dietary fat is high in calories and needs to be kept in moderation or eliminated from our diet. We fear it's dietary fat that has made us fat. The truth is that dietary fat leaves you feeling satisfied. It also helps you burn more body fat. And as long as you consume high-quality dietary fats in the quantities that you can reasonably consume in nature, they won't make you obese.

Many Americans who put forth a lot of effort trying to eat healthy and manage their weight make big mistakes when it comes to dietary fat. For example, a typical dieter will go on a diet focused on caloric restriction and will severely limit or eliminate all dietary fat. They'll order a salad with a variety of vegetables and low-fat boneless skinless chicken breast, topped with fat free raspberry vinaigrette dressing. The fiber from the vegetables will leave them feeling full, the protein from the chicken breasts will give them energy, but there's nothing to make them feel satisfied. So they end up eating bread or chips or even chocolate in an attempt to fulfill this need. The problem is that this salad is just too low in fat and calories. Instead, you should order either a higher healthy fat protein source, like grass-fed beef, salmon or tuna, or add healthy fats like nuts, avocado, or a little goat cheese to your salad. For example, take a typical guy who feels like he can't get full or satisfied without starch and feed him an eight-ounce grass-fed sirloin steak with creamed spinach. I guarantee he'll feel full from the fiber in the spinach and satisfied from the dietary fat in the steak and the cream.

Moreover, diets too low in fat may be responsible for stubborn abdominal, thigh, and butt body fat. Dieters trying to slim down by following extremely low-fat diets may be causing the exact opposite results. Researchers say that eating healthy dietary fat is an ideal way to kick-start fat-burning.

Here are a couple tips when it comes to picking the right fats:

- Healthy fats include extra virgin olive oil, organic virgin coconut oil, fish oils, flax seed oil, golden flax seeds, chia or salba seeds, most nuts and avocado.
- Avoid hydrogenated fats, partially hydrogenated oils and trans-fatty acids.
- Ensure your daily nutrition consists of enough omega-3 fatty acids. Supplement with fish or flax seed oil.

The typical Western diet is overloaded with omega-6 fatty acids and contains insufficient omega-3 fatty acids. The current ratio of omega-6 to omega-3 fatty acids in a typical U.S. diet is about 10:1, whereas in hunter-gatherer diets it is closer to 2:1. According to Paleolithic expert Dr. Loren Cordain, this dietary imbalance in fatty acids (excessive omega-6 and insufficient omega-3) is a fundamental underlying cause of many chronic diseases, including cardiovascular disease, many cancers, most inflammatory diseases, and many psychological disturbances.

Quite possibly the healthiest omega-6 source comes from the oil found in coconut. Yes, coconut oil is a saturated fat, but this is a good thing. A recent study revealed that saturated fats like coconut oil are actually healthier than polyunsaturated fats like soybean oil.

Coconut oil has become overwhelmingly popular among natural health food experts, and there are now multiple brands available at nearly every health food store. As a saturated fat, coconut oil is incredibly stable and not prone to rancidity. In fact, coconut oil that has been extracted from mature coconut meat is one of best oils to use in high-temperature cooking, as the saturated fatty acids are inert and least likely to use up antioxidants and produce free radicals. The fat in coconut meat is a source of pure energy.

One of the many benefits of coconut oil is its usefulness in reducing body fat. It contains short and medium-chain fatty acids that help in taking off excessive body fat. It's also easy to digest and helps in the healthy functioning of the thyroid and enzyme systems. Further, it increases the body's metabolism by removing stress on the pancreas, thereby burning more energy and helping you lose body fat. This is why people living in tropical coastal areas who eat coconut oil daily as their primary cooking oil are historically lean and fit.

Key takeaways from this chapter:

- **The truth about protein:**
  Sustained energy
  Muscle building and sparing
  Building blocks of every cell in your body
  It's what you absorb that counts
  You are what you eat

- **The truth about sugar:**
  Energy spikes, then crashes

Stored in fat cells

Not the ideal fuel source

An addictive drug

- **The truth about fiber:**

  Promotes healthy bowel movements

  Keeps you from overeating

  Leaves you full

- **The truth about starch:**

  Turns into sugar rapidly in the body

  Adequate amounts found in certain veggies

  Most high-starch foods make you fat

- **The truth about dietary fat:**

  Satiates you

  Body's preferred energy source

  Helps burn body fat

Chapter 8

Pre-Workout and Post-Workout Recovery Nutrition

What you consume before and after your workout can make or break not only your performance in the gym, but your results

Pre-Workout Nutrition

Champions understand that not only is the quality of what you eat fundamentally important for your health and your performance, but the timing of meals is equally imperative. While the average person only needs to think in terms of breakfast, lunch, dinner, and snacks, champions must additionally think in terms of pre- and post-workout recovery nutrition. Although some teens are beginning to recognize the importance of post-workout recovery nutrition and the small anabolic window for recovery and repair, pre-workout nutrition is typically neglected. Most youth either work out on an empty stomach or whatever they happen to have eaten on their way to the gym. Others turn to highly caffeinated sodas or "energy" drinks for a pre-workout boost. What you consume before your workout can make or break not only your performance in the gym, but your results.

Let's get back to the analogy of the multimillion-dollar high-performance race car. What would happen if someone accidentally put regular unleaded gasoline, or even a gallon of soda, into the gas tank before a big race? The high-performance car would quickly break down and not be able to perform. The same applies to your body if you show up to practice, a workout, or a game inadequately fueled. You may or may not feel lethargic depending on whether or not you've had any stimulants like caffeine, but the true consequences will show in your performance and your long-term results.

If you exercise on an empty stomach, your body will not have adequate muscle glycogen (stored carbohydrates in the muscle cells) or glycogen in the bloodstream to push you through an intense workout. Without adequate protein in your body, your body will begin to break down hard-earned muscle as fuel. You also won't be able to work out as long or as hard if you're hungry. Eating before a workout leads to sustained energy with better strength and faster recovery. It also ensures you maintain adequate blood-sugar levels so that you don't feel dizzy or nauseous, and keeps you focused on the workout rather than hunger pangs.

Pre-workout nutrition varies based on the time of day that you exercise or have practice. For example, if you are training in the early morning, you should have an easily digestible breakfast one to two hours before working out. If you are exercising in the early afternoon or evening, then your pre-workout nutrition should be a healthy meal one to two hours before your workout, including any supplements you might be taking.

Protein a few hours before a workout not only provides sustained energy throughout your workout, it also provides an anti-catabolic (muscle-sparing) effect. This means that when you are lifting weights, the protein in your system will keep you from utilizing muscle as a fuel source and help build and repair muscle cells. Your best options are complete protein sources like lean beef, fish, chicken or eggs. If you are consuming your pre-workout nutrition less than sixty minutes before your workout, choose an easier-to-digest protein source, such as FIT 365® or other high-quality, whey protein-based shakes.

In addition to protein for pre-workout nutrition, it is important to tailor the source and quantity of carbohydrates you consume to the type of sport or workout you will be performing. For example, pre-workout nutrition for a distance runner should begin the night before a big run and consist of high-carbohydrate, high-starch vegetables like spaghetti squash, acorn squash, sweet potatoes or yams. Ironically, these same types of carbohydrates are also beneficial for a football lineman looking to bulk up while maintaining good strength and energy on the playing field. However, a lightweight wrestler or a track sprinter's pre-workout nutrition before lifting weights should consist of more fast-releasing carbohydrates, like a piece of fruit—an apple or an orange—thirty minutes before going into the weight room.

Make sure you don't eat too much food, heavy food, or too many carbohydrates before you work out. Your mom was actually right when she said not to swim with a full stomach. If you eat too close to your workout or consume too many carbohydrates right before your workout, your digestive system will be competing with your muscles for the blood flow required to metabolize the food you just ate and get the workout pump you desire.

A few examples of easy pre-workout nutrition for young athletes:

- Apple with almond butter, raw honey, and coconut flakes

- Unsweetened apple chips

- Perfect Foods® bars

- Hardboiled eggs

- Organic yogurts

- FIT 365® shakes

Post-Workout Recovery Nutrition

It's not what you digest but what you absorb that counts

Many teens give it their all in the gym with dreams of building muscle and burning fat. Yet their naiveté leads to self-sabotage when they neglect the most vital component. Muscle is not built and fat is not lost in the gym; these changes are made after you leave the gym through proper nutritional choices. Many athletes ruin their program by poorly refueling. They either rationalize that exercise allows them to eat whatever they want or they neglect one of the most important meals of the day: the post workout recovery meal. Within thirty minutes to an hour of working out, your body has an anabolic (muscle-building) and anti-catabolic (muscle-sparing) window where you can capitalize on optimal gains. In order to achieve the highest yield on your workout investment, your body requires six different nutrients: quality protein, quality carbohydrates and dietary oils, quality water, electrolytes, and enzymes.

Top six concerns in a post-workout recovery drink:

1. **Quality protein**

   Biological Value (BV) refers to how well and how quickly your body can actually use the protein you consume. According to Dr. David Williams, whey protein is the new standard score of 100, egg scores a 93.7, milk protein scores an 84.5, soy protein scores a 72.8, and rice protein scores a 64.0. [15]

   It is becoming common knowledge that whey is superior to other proteins for post-workout recovery drinks. Yet not all whey protein is the same. In the case of whey protein, grass-fed whey protein is far superior to commercial whey protein isolates and concentrates. Nearly all whey protein products are a processed, isolated or concentrated by-product from grain and soy-fed cows that are pumped full of hormones and antibiotics. Instead, choose a native whey protein from a grass-fed cow, as it will be more beneficial for rapid tissue repair, muscle building, and immune support. It's glutamine rich and high in Branch Chain Amino Acids (BCAAs) and fat-burning CLA. [16]

2. **Quality carbohydrates**

   Post exercise, your muscles are the most susceptible to storing glycogen (sugar). Any carbohydrates you ingest that are not burned as fuel or stored in the muscle cells will be stored as body fat. Small amounts of carbohydrates from fruit are the best call. On the other hand, standard recommendations like maltodextrin (grain-based starch) or 75 grams of dextrose are poor choices if you are trying to lose body fat while gaining muscle.

3. **Quality oils**

Healthy dietary oils work better than carbohydrates as fuel. Their cholesterol is needed as a precursor to all your natural anabolic hormones. Without cholesterol, we can't make many hormones, including testosterone, estrogen, pregnenolone, or DHEA, in our bodies. You need to have high enough levels of cholesterol in your body to manufacture optimal quantities of these fat-burning, muscle-building hormones.

4. **Quality water**

Proper hydration after exercise is essential. That's the beauty of a post-workout recovery drink: you are able to ingest quality nutrients and properly rehydrate simultaneously. You should drink roughly one ounce for every pound of body weight.

5. **Electrolytes**

Vital minerals like potassium and sodium are essential for post-workout recovery, as they are lost while sweating. Many sea salts are rich in minerals that your body needs, such as sodium, potassium, calcium, and magnesium. Unlike highly processed table salt, these minerals don't cause kidney and adrenal stress. Coconut water is your best choice for replacing electrolytes lost during your workout.

6. **Enzymes**

It's not what you digest but what you absorb that counts. Digestive enzymes will break down the ingredients into nutrients that your body can readily digest and more efficiently absorb.

Key takeaways from this chapter:

Champions understand that not only is the quality of what you eat fundamentally important for your health and your performance, but the timing of meals is equally essential.

In addition to protein for pre-workout nutrition, it is important to tailor the source and quantity of carbohydrates you consume to the type of sport and workout you will be performing.

A few examples of easy pre-workout nutrition for youth:

- Apple with almond butter, raw honey, and coconut flakes

- Unsweetened apple chips

- Perfect Foods® bars

- Hardboiled eggs

- Organic yogurts

Top six concerns in a post-workout recovery drink:

- Quality protein

- Quality carbohydrates

- Quality oils

- Quality water

- Electrolytes

- Enzymes

Chapter 9

Water Is Nature's Energy Drink

The secrets of the best fat burner and performance enhancer on the market

I constantly have both teens and adults coming to me looking for the competitive edge. They want a little magic pill or energy drink that will increase their energy, improve their stamina, and give them ultimate fat-burning. Sadly, such a solution doesn't exist. The answer doesn't come in a pill—it actually comes in a liquid. And it's free! Water is the fountain of youth and nature's most important substance for energy and weight management.

According to naturopath Dr. Dave Carpenter, optimal hydration is vital to your health, fitness and performance because water performs the following functions:

- Stabilization of body temperature
- Removal of lactic acid and waste products from muscle cells, which helps dissolve minerals and other nutrients, making them accessible to the body
- Facilitation of the reactions in the cell mitochondria that release energy from the energy currency molecule, known as ATP
- Transport of nutrients and oxygen to cells throughout the body

Moreover, water helps alkalize your body, as it detoxifies and removes acid waste.

The biggest reason why water is the best fat burner on the planet is that it suppresses your appetite while it speeds up your metabolism.

DEHYDRATION

Our primary fuel as humans is a combination of water and minerals. We can survive days without food but we cannot last much more than 100 hours without water. [17]

Frequently, when you're feeling hungry, you may just be thirsty, and by the time you feel thirsty you're already dehydrated. And the small amount of water required to quench your thirst is generally not enough to hydrate the body. It only takes a slight dehydration to reduce your energy levels and performance and alter your ability to think clearly.

Most teens underestimate the amount of water lost during exercise. The loss of one and one half quarts of water, a common amount for teens to lose during a workout, results in a 25% loss in stamina. Keep in mind that our bodies are more than 70% water. Our blood is more than 85% water, our muscles more than 75% water, and our liver is 96% water.[18]

Dehydration is one of the main reasons it can take so long for teens to recover from intense workouts. Proper hydration reduces recovery time and enhances performance. Just a 5% drop in body fluids can cause a 25 to 30% loss of energy. If you're 1% dehydrated, it can cause a 5% decrease in cognitive function. Fortunately, when you chug down a glass or two of water your hydration and energy levels can improve quickly. [17] A good rule of thumb is to drink one ounce of water for every pound of body weight. It's helpful to carry a liter-sized water bottle with you throughout the day. Dehydration can lead to headaches. Drink a big glass of water right when you wake up in the morning to help you rehydrate after sleeping.

Remember, water you get in a public water fountain can fall short of the quality of water your body needs. Make sure your water is at least filtered of environmental toxins like herbicides and pesticides, like mountain spring water or water from another untainted source. But if you only have access to a public fountain, it's still a much better choice than not drinking enough water.

ENERGY DRINKS

The pressure facing teens to perform at their best, both in school and in sports, typically leads to high stress and a lack of quality sleep. For a quick fix, an overwhelming amount of teens reach for an energy drink to help them make it through the day or to get them "pumped up" before practice or a workout.

The energy drink business has exploded into a multibillion-dollar industry. Unfortunately, most energy drinks are simply sugar, chemicals and an obscene amount of caffeine. For example, the average soft drink contains 30 mg of caffeine and a typical cup of coffee contains 80 mg, yet some energy drinks contain 200 mg or more of caffeine! Worst of all, many young athletes guzzle down two or more of these energy drinks daily. While the FDA regulates the amount of caffeine in soft drinks—allowing a maximum of 72 mg of caffeine per 12-ounce serving (6 mg/oz.)—it hasn't yet regulated the caffeine content in energy drinks.[19]

What the caffeine and other stimulants in these energy drinks do is leave you mentally wired but physically exhausted underneath it all. And the caffeine jolt is short lived. While a typical "caffeine buzz" lasts only a few hours, the biological half-life of caffeine—the time required for the body to eliminate one half of the total amount of caffeine—is roughly five hours for adults and can be more than double that in children. [20] This means that if you have an energy drink after school, your body will still be dealing with the caffeine effects late into the night. Not only will this diminish your quality of sleep and your immune system, but it could also hinder your performance and mental alertness.

While some caffeine may be beneficial, the quantity of caffeine—let alone the absurd amount of sugar in a typical energy drink—can be detrimental to your health and your performance. But don't think choosing a sugar- and calorie-free energy drink is a better option. Considering a calorie is a unit of energy, calorie-free is frankly impossible. If it's truly "calorie-free," then what are you putting in your body? Just a thought.

COFFEE

Lately it seems that coffee shops are popping up on every corner. Have you ever been to a coffee shop in the early afternoon?

Surprisingly, you'll probably find them filled with kids looking for that afternoon boost. While market analysis firms don't track coffee consumption for youths under eighteen, the percentage of eighteen to twenty-four-year-olds who drink coffee every day doubled from 2003 to 2007, going from 16 to 31%, according to the National Coffee Association. Yet the Food and Drug Administration doesn't provide any recommendations on caffeine consumption for adolescents. The American Dietetic Association doesn't, either, but at least gives some guidelines. Between 200 and 300 milligrams a day—about two to three cups of coffee—is safe for adults. Typically, the coffee drinks that are appealing to teens are loaded with sugar and fat. While the average soft drink has 150 calories, many coffee drinks are 300 to 400 calories, which is close to the total recommended calories for a meal. All of these drinks are low-nutrient drinks that can easily sabotage your fat loss and health goals.

SODA

New research points to soft drinks as the leading cause of childhood obesity. You need to eliminate nearly all soda, especially diet soda, from your diet completely! Among the many harmful substances in diet soda, they contain the artificial sweetener aspartame, phosphoric acid and carbonation that depletes calcium from your bones. Aspartame in diet sodas is also responsible for weight gain. The sweet taste of diet soda creates a cephalic phase response, which causes the liver to prepare to receive sugar. When no sugar appears, the liver prompts the body to eat, which can result in increased hunger and overeating. The cephalic phase response also triggers the release of insulin, which stores sugar in the bloodstream. When you consume aspartame, you raise your insulin levels and cause the sugar in your blood to be converted into fat. Older fat is not metabolized. [21]

Again, these same people are not aware of secret #1. They feel if they drink diet sodas and calorie-free energy drinks they won't gain weight. Yet the evidence shows otherwise. An eight-year study performed at University of Texas Health Science Center showed that the risk of being overweight soared by 41% for every can or bottle of diet soft drink a person consumed each day. The risk of becoming overweight grew from 36.5% for up to a half a can a day to 47.2% for more than two cans each day. Ironically, this is lower than the rate for regular soft drink consumers. A typical teen consumes two 12-ounce soft drinks per day, accounting for 300 empty calories and 20 teaspoons of sugar at 20% of the teen's daily caloric intake. [22]

COCONUT WATER: NATURE'S ULTIMATE SPORTS DRINK

The secret elixir out of the South Pacific, coconut water, has finally transferred over to the mainstream and is gaining major ground in the sports drink community. Coconut water is referred to as nature's isotonic sports drink because it contains the same balanced concentrations of electrolytes as our blood in far superior amounts to manufactured sports drinks, and without all of the unnecessary sugar.

According to Mortin Satin, chief of the United Nations' Food and Agriculture Organization, "Coconut water is the very stuff of nature, biologically pure, full of natural sugars, salts, and vitamins to ward off fatigue... and is the next wave of energy drinks, but natural!"

Compared to manufactured sports and energy drinks, coconut water:

- Contains more potassium and less sodium
- Acts as a prebiotic by supporting beneficial bacteria in the gut
- Contains less sugar
- Contains natural vitamins, minerals, protein, and lauric acid, a healthy nutrient present in human mothers' milk
- Has a higher nutrient concentration than orange juice with less calories and sugar
- Contains more chloride, a chemical the human body needs for metabolism (the process of turning food into energy)
- Speeds up your metabolism, which can aid in weight loss
- Alkalizes your body to help balance the pH in your blood

Remember, athletes perspire far more than sedentary individuals. This serves as your body's natural cooling system to keep you from overheating. But not only do you sweat out water, your body also loses vital electrolytes. Drinking coconut water daily when exercising can help your body feel hydrated and replenish your electrolytes. [23]

Key takeaways from this chapter:

- The biggest reason why water is the best fat burner on the planet is that it suppresses your appetite while it speeds up your metabolism.
- Frequently, when you're feeling hungry, you may just be thirsty, and by the time you feel thirsty you're already dehydrated.
- The loss of one and one half quarts of water, a common amount for athletes to lose during performance, results in a 25% loss in stamina.
- The caffeine and other stimulants in energy drinks leave you mentally wired but physically exhausted underneath it all.
- New research points to soft drinks as the leading cause of childhood obesity.
- Coconut water is referred to as nature's isotonic sports drink because it contains the same balanced concentrations of electrolytes as our blood in far superior amounts to manufactured sports drinks, and without all of the unnecessary sugar.

Chapter 10

Ask Any Farmer: Excessive Grains, Sugar, and Soy Make You Sick and Overweight!

Foods that leave you frustrated, as you can't out-exercise poor nutrition

I can't begin to tell you how many aspiring young athletes have come to me after training for an endurance event like a marathon or a triathlon and actually increased body fat during the process. This shocking phenomenon is due to the high amount of processed carbohydrates from grain, sugar and soy products they are consuming in an attempt to keep higher, sustained energy levels. Many endurance athletes follow a high-processed carbohydrate diet of breads, pasta, cereals, and liquid sugary gels with a low fat intake and use incomplete protein sources like peanut butter for energy. This diet can leave frustrated athletes competing with twenty-plus unnecessary pounds on their body and at a level nowhere near their potential. Bottom line: you can't out-exercise poor nutrition.

However, if you're an endurance or a strength athlete, you may require a higher quantity of high-starch carbohydrates than our Paleolithic ancestors consumed. Unfortunately, many young athletes choose large portions of the wrong starch options to "carb-load." **Starchy vegetables should make up your primary starch servings instead of pasta, bread, or rice.** Keep away from sugar cereals, breads and starchy snack foods except during your occasional planned indulgence. And remember, starch servings are incredibly small for being so calorically dense. For example, an 80-

calorie serving of starch is half a cup mashed potatoes, a third of a cup of rice (roughly the size of a golf ball), half a cup of pasta, a slice of bread, or half a cup flaked cereal. As you know, it's nearly impossible to eat only one serving of starch at a time. Unfortunately, mainstream dietary guidelines recommend six to eleven servings of grains per day, which is up to 880 calories from grains or up to 60% of an individual's recommended daily caloric intake. This guidance has left Americans in the same condition as grain and soy-fed livestock—overweight, bloated, sick and dependent on medications like antibiotics.

The consequences of a diet based around high consumption of grains and soy are parallel between humans and livestock. So if farmers know cows are ruminants, which means they efficiently convert grass to milk or meat—and even the American Heart Association promotes eating grass-fed beef versus grain-fed beef—why would farmers feed their livestock grains and soy, which aren't as healthy as grass? The main reason is because today's average farmer is not an individual but a corporation with the objective of making as much money as possible per cow. Feeding livestock grains and soy enables them to gain weight quickly at levels they would not be able to achieve if they were pasture-fed. The factory farms sell meat by the pound, so the more an animal weighs, the more money they can generate from that livestock.

According to Paleolithic nutrition expert Dr. Loren Cordain, "It was only with the dawn of agriculture (around 10,000 years ago) that our diets evolved to include what we think of as staple foods now. DNA evidence shows that genetically, humans have hardly changed at all (to be specific, the human genome has changed less than 0.02%) in 40,000 years. This means that the genetic makeup of Paleolithic people is virtually identical to our own... Nature determined what our bodies needed thousands of years before civilization developed, before people started farming and raising domesticated livestock." [4]

Many young athletes are confused about why whole grain staple foods like whole wheat bread, brown rice, and whole grain cereals are not recommended staple foods for every meal. They're not recommended because grains cause inflammation, contain antinutrients, and rapidly turn into sugar in your body. Antinutrients are chemicals that prevent your body from absorbing healthy nutrients and can damage your gastrointestinal and immune systems. Nutritionally induced inflammation comes from eating foods that increase inflammation, which in turn may increase your muscle and joint pain and risk of chronic disease. While our Paleolithic ancestors may have died at a much younger age than we currently do, they didn't die of heart disease, diabetes, and cancer— which currently leading causes of death and are in many cases diet-related.

When comparing early agriculturalists to their hunter-gatherer ancestors, studies have revealed more infectious diseases than their ancestors, more childhood mortality, more osteoporosis and other bone mineral disorders, and countless vitamin and mineral-deficiency diseases like scurvy and iron-deficiency anemia. A diet based on grains provided the calories but lacked the vital nutrients of our nature-intended diet of lean meats, fruits and vegetables. So why did our ancestors turn from hunter-gatherers into agriculturalists? In one word: scarcity. Our free will as humans led us to settle down, build homes for our families, and stop being nomadic. Yet the rest of the animal kingdom remained nomadic: birds flocked, buffalo roamed, and fish swam. We stopped hunting our food and eating seasonal vegetables and fruits. We began cultivating grains like rice and then wheat and corn, which didn't have the issues of spoilage like fruits, vegetables, and lean meats. This led to an enormous population explosion.

For example, humans were not designed to eat bread daily, regardless of whether it's whole wheat or white bread. For nearly all cultures that consider bread a staple food, wheat was not indigenous to (naturally found in) their environment. Wheat was one of the first crops that could be easily cultivated on a large scale, and had the additional advantage of yielding a harvest that provides long-term food for storage. Wheat helped feed the masses in times of poverty and scarcity, as wheat has the ability to self-pollinate and grow almost anywhere.

What most of us don't realize is that when you consume grain products they rapidly turn into sugar in the body. Most of this low-nutrient energy is then stored in your fat cells. Moreover, sugar wreaks havoc on the human body in countless ways. We are abusing sugar to the point that it is slowly killing us. **Sugar, especially in the form of high fructose corn syrup, is the single largest source of calories in the American diet.** In 1700, the average person consumed about 4 pounds of sugar per year. In 1800, the average person consumed about 18 pounds of sugar per year. In 1900, the average person had consumed 90 pounds of sugar per year. Today, the average consumption has soared to 180 pounds of sugar per year! Sugar contributes to obesity, compromised immune systems, hyperactivity, depression, anxiety, premature aging, diabetes, and many other conditions. [20]

Here are five potential side effects of consuming too much sugar that you may not know about:

- Sugar feeds cancer cells and has been connected with the development of cancer of the breast, ovaries, prostate, rectum, pancreas, biliary tract, lung, gallbladder and stomach. [21]
- Decreasing sugar intake can increase emotional stability. [22]
- Your body changes sugar into two to five times more fat in the bloodstream than it does starch. [23]
- Sugar can cause a rapid rise of adrenaline, hyperactivity, anxiety, difficulty concentrating, and crankiness in children. [24]
- Sugar can reduce learning capacity, adversely affect grades and cause learning disorders. [25]

A high-sugar diet can be far more dangerous than a diet high in fat. Most people don't realize how much added sugar is in what they consume—especially in diet and fat-free processed foods. Worst of all, most Americans don't worry about side effects of their actions or disease until it's too late. Typically, teens age twelve to seventeen feel invincible, as if nothing bad could possibly happen to them; they're mostly interested in the present. If they don't feel the negative side effects of something immediately, future ramifications for their actions and behaviors are an afterthought. This can cause them to engage in high-risk behaviors as they try to become independent. It is not until eighteen to twenty-one that teens begin to realize their mortality and begin to worry about the future. Some still think they are invincible, but this wanes. Yet the correlation between nutrition, fitness, and longevity doesn't typically become a priority until they reach their late twenties to early thirties—and by then, poor habits have already been ingrained and are nearly impossible to break.

Now, I am not suggesting that you have to eliminate all grain products and sugar completely from your healthy lifestyle nutritional plan. However, you need to change how you view them. These are not staple foods to be eaten all day every day, but occasional indulgences that fit both your need for convenience and your desire for a treat, like some pasta or a slice of pizza. Remember, you'll only need a small amount of grain to satisfy these desires, and all of your meals that include grains should also include adequate quantities of lean meat, vegetables and healthy oils. And when you choose grains products, reach for the least processed sources, such as amaranth, barley, basmati rice, black beans, brown rice, couscous, garbanzo beans, steel-cut oats, pinto beans, quinoa, rye, spelt or wild rice.

Key takeaways from this chapter:

- Current nutritional guidance on grains and soy has left Americans in the same condition as grain and soy-fed livestock—overweight, bloated, sick, and dependent on medications like antibiotics.

- What most of us don't realize is that when you consume grain products they rapidly turn into sugar in the body.
- Sugar can cause a rapid rise of adrenaline, hyperactivity, anxiety, difficulty concentrating, and crankiness in children.
- You'll only need a small amount of grain to satisfy your desires, and all of your meals that include grains should also include adequate quantities of lean meat, vegetables and healthy oils.

Chapter 11

The Manipulated Food Chain: You Are What You Eat
Nutrition facts panels only tell part of the story

Every living thing requires energy to live. Food chains show how each living thing gets food, and how nutrients and energy are passed from creature to creature. It all begins with plant life, as plants use sunlight, water and nutrients to get energy in a process called photosynthesis. Herbivores eat these plants for energy and we human beings, as omnivores, get our energy from eating a combination of these plants and eating the animals that eat plants, as well as their by-products, including milk, cheese and eggs. But what if human beings get in the way of Mother Nature and manipulate the food chain? How does this change the makeup of the animals we eat and affect our health and performance in the gym?

I'm sure we all learned about food chains in high school biology class. For example, man eats cow and cow eats grass. But in 2012, that's not the way food chains work in the commercial food industry. Nowadays, a typical commercial food chain looks more like this: man eats cow, cow eats corn and soy, antibiotics, hormones, other drugs, and, up until recently, other cows' parts. And commercial chickens and farm-raised fish have essentially the same problem. [26]

In nature, chickens aren't vegetarians; they're omnivores. The ideal chicken is free-range, eating numerous bugs and wild plants and consuming 30% of their calories from grass. Unfortunately, farmed fish are also fed corn, for the first time in history introducing omega-

6 fatty acids into the ocean's food chains. The entire ocean food chain is based on single-celled green plankton, which is the "grass" of the sea. Plankton has no seeds, so all wild seafood has only omega-3 fats. (27)

There are two main kinds of fatty acids: omega-3 and omega-6. Omega-3s come from the green parts of plants, while omega-6s come from the seeds of plants. We need approximately equal amounts of omega-3s and omega-6s in our bodies. But because of practices feeding livestock corn and soy instead of grass, we are consuming huge proportions of omega-6 and very little omega-3. Meat and dairy products from animals fed a high-grain diet have up to ten times more omega-6s than products from grass-fed animals. Consuming high levels of omega-6 raises our "bad cholesterol," and keeps our "good cholesterol" low. Consuming equal amounts of omega-3s and omega-6s raises good cholesterol and lowers bad cholesterol.

Why is it so important to eat animals that eat what nature intended? According to the most comprehensive analysis to date, grass-fed beef is better for human health than grain-fed beef in ten different ways. A joint effort study in 2009 between the United States Department of Agriculture (USDA) and researchers at Clemson University compared grain-fed beef to grass-fed beef and found that grass-fed beef was lower in total fat, higher in beta-carotene, higher in vitamin E (alpha-tocopherol), higher in the B-vitamins thiamin and riboflavin, higher in the minerals calcium, magnesium, and potassium, higher in total omega-3s, healthier in ratio of omega-6 to omega-3 fatty acids (1.65 vs. 4.84), higher in CLA (cis-9 trans-11), a potential cancer fighter, higher in vaccenic acid (which can be transformed into CLA), and lower in the saturated fats linked with heart disease.

How does the makeup of food affect us? Most people think protein is protein, carbs are carbs, fat is fat, and calories are calories, and all that matters is the calorie count and the grams of protein, carbs and fat in a particular food. The truth is that nutrition fact panels only tell part of the story and explain nothing about the quality of the food you're eating. A recent study showed that mice fed the same amount of omega-6 fatty acids present in the modern Western diet grow fatter and fatter with each succeeding generation and have the warning signs of diabetes, versus mice that eat a healthy balance of omega-6 and omega-3 with equal amounts of exercise [28]. This study suggests that if we switch to food with a healthy balance of omega-6 and omega-3 fatty acids, we will be leaner and healthier. It just goes to show that French researcher Gerard Aihaud was right when he said, "Omega-6 is like a fat-producing bomb..."

Nature's Food Chain:

Man (consumes) —> Grass-Fed Cow (consumes) —> Grass and Other Foliage

Man (consumes) —> Free-Range Chicken (consumes) —> Bugs and Wild Plants

Man (consumes) —> Wild Fish (consumes) —> Small Wild Fish or Sea Life/Algae

Modern-Day Commercial Food Chain:

Man (consumes) —> Corn-Fed Cow (consumes) —> Corn, Soy, Antibiotics and Hormones

Man (consumes) —> Farm-Raised Chicken (consumes) —> Corn, Soy, and Antibiotics

Man (consumes) —> Farm-Raised Fish (consumes) —> Corn

Key takeaways from this chapter:

- Food chains show how each living thing gets food, and how nutrients and energy are passed from creature to creature.
- Nowadays, a typical commercial food chain looks like this: man eats cow, cow eats corn and soy, antibiotics, hormones, other drugs, and, up until recently, other cows' parts. And commercial chickens and farm-raised fish have essentially the same problem.
- Grass-fed beef is far superior to grain-fed beef, as a new study suggests that if we switch to food with a healthy balance of omega-6 and omega-3 fatty acids (like grass-fed beef), we will be leaner and healthier.

Chapter 12

Supplement Pros and Scams

Why we need supplements and what supplements every young athlete should take

It's not always easy or practical to maintain perfect nutrition all the time. Supplementation builds upon the foundation of proper nutrition to ensure daily requirements are met. Since we don't eat fruit off the tree or raw meat anymore, we lose micronutrients and critical enzymes in the cooking and storing process.

According to the *Nutrition Business Journal*, Americans spend $15.6 billion each year on nutritional supplements. The major problem for most teens is that they get confused by hearing so many different perspectives on supplementation—from either reading muscle magazines or talking with friends who have read these magazines. The secret is that supplement companies produce most of these magazines. So what you believe is an unbiased report or article on the effectiveness of a particular supplement is actually a paid advertisement.

Moreover, since young athletes are not properly educated on proper nutrition and supplementation, many use a "shotgun" approach to supplementation. This approach means that they will take a multitude of supplements at the same time with no regulation of dosage or consideration of how these supplements interact with one another. With the FDA's hands-off approach to supplements, many teens are creating their own cocktail of supplements to make themselves bigger, stronger and wired, with no supervision over their actions. A good rule of thumb when it comes to supplements is that if a supplement makes you extremely wired or jittery, let alone makes your heart race, and if you cannot get the ingredients from real food, you shouldn't put it in your body.

The supplements I recommend for athletes and non-athletes alike are high-potency nutrients that complement a healthy nutritional lifestyle. Too many teens fall victim to the marketing propaganda of supplement companies that a miracle pill/powder that will turn them into Superman or Wonder Woman without hard work in the gym or a healthy diet. Truth is, behind all of the smoke and mirrors, the models that are hired to represent these products are doing so much more than simply taking whatever supplement they're endorsing. Many of them are using steroids and other hormones to get their bodies into what is referred to as "contest shape," and excessive exercise is a huge part of their lifestyle and required for their profession. Moreover, these models or spokespeople don't maintain this shape year-round. Your goal should be to maintain a healthy lifestyle 365 days a year so you are always able to perform at your best.

While everybody has different supplemental requirements, there are a few foundational supplements that will benefit anyone regardless of their fitness level. It is wise to always consult a physician before you take any new supplements.

- **Omega 3 Fatty Acids**—These are healthy fats found in fish, grass-fed beef, walnuts and flaxseed. Throughout history, people around the world ate a ratio of about two-to-one omega-6-to-omega-3 fats. This created a healthy balance of fats, which allowed the body to work efficiently. The shift to processed, convenient foods has brought the typical American diet to a ratio of up to twenty-to-one, meaning most Americans eat up to twenty times more omega-6 fats than omega-3. This imbalance is thought to contribute to a host of diseases, including heart disease, arthritis and many types of cancer. The best supplemental sources are krill oil, cod liver oil and flaxseed oil. Omega-3s have been clinically proven to help lower cholesterol levels, fight depression, reduce inflammation, improve cardiovascular health, and much more.

- **Multi-vitamin Multi-mineral** — Since our soil and food are depleted of quality vitamins and minerals, taking a quality multi will protect against a multitude of diseases, reduce premature aging of cells, strengthen your organs, and much more. Choose a whole-food-based multi-vitamin and mineral, as it is sourced from real foods instead of a typical synthetic vitamin created to mimic vitamins in their natural state. Also, keep away from single-pill multi-vitamins, as you can't fit all of the quality vitamins and minerals you need into one pill. Water-soluble vitamins need to be taken multiple times per day.

- **B & C Vitamin Packets**—Vitamins B & C are water-soluble vitamins that are depleted from your bloodstream increasingly by stress. Benefits include increased energy levels, immune system enhancement and more.

- **Probiotics**—80% of your immune system is located in your digestive system. Probiotics provide support for both your digestive system and your immune system. Probiotics will help you feel better and lose weight simultaneously.

- **FIT 365®**—A complete nutritional shake like FIT 365® is a perfect post-workout recovery drink or breakfast and helps meet your needs for quality grass-fed whey protein and fiber, as well as providing the fat-burning benefits of coconut oil. Make sure you avoid products with artificial ingredients, sweeteners and fillers.

- **Green Drinks**—Green drinks help alkalize the body by neutralizing the excess acids of a modern Western diet. They can help increase your energy levels and reduce your urge to snack or reach for high sugar or caffeine-based energy drinks. There are many green drinks on the market, each offering the nutritional benefits of the green plants and vegetables that are often lacking in our diets.

- **Coconut Water**—Coconut water is referred to as nature's isotonic sports drink because it contains the same balanced concentrations of electrolytes as our blood, in far superior amounts to manufactured sports drinks and without all of the unnecessary sugar. Learn more about coconut water's benefits in the chapter "Water Is Nature's Energy Drink."

- **Coconut Oil**—Coconut oil is the most delicious and best fat-burning oil on the planet! High in medium-chain fatty acids

(MCFAs) and lauric acid, coconut oil has been clinically proven to promote weight loss, provide instant energy, and support proper thyroid function. Coconut oil that has been extracted from mature coconut meat is one of the best oils to use in high-temperature cooking, as the saturated fatty acids are inert and least likely to use up antioxidants and produce free radicals. In addition, it's easy to digest and helps in healthy functioning of the enzyme systems. Coconut oil's short and medium-chain fatty acids also help take off excess body fat. It increases your metabolism by removing stress on the pancreas, thereby burning more energy and helping you lose body fat. This is why people living in tropical coastal areas who eat coconut oil daily as their primary cooking oil are historically lean and fit.

- **Psyllium Seed Husk or Flaxseed Fiber**—According to the American Dietetic Association, adults should consume between 20 and 35 grams of fiber per day. However, the average American consumes only 12 to 15 grams. In contrast, people in China consume as much as 77 grams of fiber per day. For youth up to age eighteen, the recommended daily dose (in grams) is determined by adding five to a child's age. For example, a thirteen-year-old needs 18 grams of fiber a day. Dietary fibers are shown to support cardiac and gastrointestinal health, immune function, and weight management. Psyllium seed husks are indigestible in human beings and are used as a regular dietary supplement to improve and maintain regular GI transit. Fiber and fiber-rich foods help regulate blood sugar, control hunger, and enhance the feeling of fullness—these are all essential to losing weight and keeping it off.

Conditional Supplements for Certain High School Athletes:

- **Caffeine**—Once you reach high school and have been exercising for a few years, a small quantity of caffeine from a cup of coffee or green tea may be beneficial, as it promotes increased focus, intensity and energy. But remember, the energy benefits you will receive from the nutrients above are far superior to any short-term benefit of caffeine.

- **Covalent Bonded Glutamine**—For certain athletes who are incorporating heavier resistance training and high-intensity cardio workouts, Glutamine could serve as a useful supplement. This is different than the free-form amino acid L-Glutamine, as it delivers up to ten times more glutamine to the bloodstream. Glutamine is an amino acid, one of the building blocks of protein. It's the most abundant amino acid in our body, and highly concentrated in our muscles. Glutamine has recently been reclassified as a conditionally essential amino acid. This means that while the body can make glutamine, there are times when the body's need for glutamine is greater than its ability to produce it. Studies have shown glutamine can increase protein synthesis (which leads to increased muscle mass), improve immune system function, increase nitrogen retention, decrease muscle breakdown, and decrease recovery time needed after a workout.

Key takeaways from this chapter:

Supplementation builds upon the foundation of proper nutrition to ensure daily requirements are met.

The supplements I recommend for athletes and non-athletes alike are high-potency nutrients that complement the healthy nutritional lifestyle of an athlete.

There are a few foundational supplements that will benefit anyone regardless of their sport. It is wise to always consult a physician before you take any new supplements.

- Omega-3 fatty acids
- Multi-vitamin multi-mineral
- B & C vitamin packets
- Probiotics
- FIT 365®
- Green drinks
- Coconut water
- Coconut oil
- Psyllium seed husk or flaxseed fiber

Conditional Supplements for Certain High School Athletes:

- Caffeine
- Covalent Bonded Glutamine

Chapter 13

Train with a Purpose
Why failing to plan is planning to fail

Whether you want to sculpt a lean and fit body or become a better athlete, we all have a rough idea of where we want to be, but we need a game plan to get there. Once you've decided to turn these secrets into lifestyle habits, it's time to create a game plan that's clear and easy to follow.

When I was in seventh grade, I sat down with my mom's friend, who was a teacher, and she taught me how to set short and long-term goals, how to schedule, and how to develop a game plan. We spent hours working on organizational skills. We charted out my typical day to ensure I was able to fit in all of my homework around school and practice, that I had time for all of my other responsibilities, like chores and my newspaper route, and that I was even able to fit in TV time and time for simply being a kid.

Afterward, we developed some short and long-term goals. These goals needed to be specific and achievable. She taught me not to be afraid to aim high, and suggested I set some long-term goals that were achievable if I put forth the hard work. For instance, athletically, I set short-term goals of working on my vertical jump for twenty minutes five days per week, lifting weights at least three days per week, and playing basketball every day. Two of my long-term athletic goals were to dunk a basketball and be able to bench press 300 pounds. My short-term goals were processes to help me achieve my long-term visions. And by implementing this game plan, I was not only able to achieve all of these goals, I blew them out of the water! It took me longer than anticipated, but by the time I was 21, I could dunk a basketball with ease, had benched 375 pounds for two repetitions, had played college water polo, and had competed in a national qualifying bodybuilding competition. None of these accomplishments came easy, as I am not genetically gifted for athletics. However, I had spent years working on my health and fitness, and hard work pays off. Best of all, it never felt like work, as I found ways to make the process fun. Living a healthy lifestyle became my life's passion. Now, my passion has now become my career.

Just like when I was a kid, you need to develop an action plan so that every time you go into the gym you'll know what you're doing and can focus on intensity and productivity. Simply being there won't get you in shape. You need to know what your workouts will look like. That's why initially working out with a trainer or a coach is so important. Ideally, you'll want to have an action plan that will change as your body gets used to it.

It's not about how long you spend in the gym but intensity and productivity. Your goal should be the amount of work you can get done in the most efficient time and in the most effective manner. The scene in a typical high school weight room is many kids socializing, goofing off with no real plan of action except to "get big." There's no adhering to scientific principles of time under tension or focus on what muscles they're trying to work or movement patterns they're trying to complete. Intensity is nominal at best, and vision for what these kids are trying to achieve is lacking.

However, champions walk into the gym confident and determined. They know exactly what they're there to do and how each workout fits into the big picture of achieving their goals. They train with a purpose.

Before you even step into the gym, you need to develop a game plan. This game plan involves the principles of strategy, benchmarking, and execution and is devised before you go to the gym to help you achieve your goals.

- **Strategy**—Gathering the proper facts and preparing a plan of action. This includes analyzing your current status, such as body composition, scale weight, physical capabilities and limitations.
- **Benchmarking**—Measuring your current performance against your past condition to gauge success.
- **Execution**—Making the conditions work for you. This involves scheduling, preparation and follow-through.

Let's compare these principles to your schoolwork. Would you be successful in school if instead of studying the course material you based your exam answers on what you saw on TV or read in a magazine? Would you get into the college of your dreams without a concrete plan of action? I doubt it. Yet most of us succumb to quick schemes such as "melt away the fat in your sleep." People find it hard to believe, in this age of scientific breakthroughs and medical miracles, that an effortless fitness and weight-loss method doesn't exist. But it doesn't. These are all advertising gimmicks that play on our emotions. It takes unleashing your own I.F. Factor—your internal fortitude—to achieve a healthy body and live the championship lifestyle.

According to Brian Grasso , founder of the International Youth Fitness Association, there are three different training classifications for youths, depending on the age of a kid. From age six to nine, the goal is guided discovery. From age ten to thirteen, the goal is learning exploration. And from age fourteen and up, the goal is to train with application. Guided discovery consists of simply having fun with multi-directional movement-based drills like running, climbing, crawling, skipping and jumping. The exploration phase is the perfect time to start learning skills. It's still fun, organized play, but kids can begin to perform more complex skills as they focus on form, like squatting, throwing and kicking, changing speed and direction. Lastly, during the application phase, it's time to train with direction and begin adding resistance in the form of dumbbells, kettlebells and other forms of functional training equipment. In all three phases, it's important that the kids enjoy what they're doing.

You need to ensure that your program not only meets the demands of your health and fitness goals or your sport but, most importantly, is based around having fun and positive reinforcement. For example, if you are too hard on yourself and stop enjoying the process, you will quickly get burnt out and lose your passion for play. This is exactly why the mentality of working out needs to become "funning out" and fitness and sports need to get back to the root idea of playing for the love of the game. **Too many times, the passion for simply playing the game is sucked right out of kids due to the intense focus on the outcome of winning versus the enjoyment of playing.**

Once you get to high school age, everything begins to change. This is the age group where training with a purpose becomes vitally important. While strength-based athletes like football players and wrestlers are well aware of the benefits of resistance training as part of their game plan, many young endurance athletes frown upon lifting weights because they fear it will make them too bulky and slow them down. Still others believe it's beneficial as long as it involves low weight and high repetitions. The truth is neither of these statements is correct. Whether or not resistance training is beneficial for endurance athletes is more about having a sport-specific game plan than anything else.

During any endurance sport, you're contracting your muscles at low to moderate force thousands of times over. Resistance training, especially strength and power training, involves the polar opposite: high intensity and high force output for a short duration. On paper, it would seem that intermingling the two types of training would be of no benefit—or even counterproductive. Yet modern science has proven that implementing resistance training programs into endurance athlete training protocols can be highly effective as long as periodization and specificity are taken into consideration.

Specificity refers to ensuring your program is customized to your unique needs. Many people think performing two sets of 15 to 20 repetitions using light to moderate weights is best for fat loss as well as endurance athletes. However, this type of training does not condition the neuromuscular system for long-distance events. Conversely, strength training should be the foundation of any endurance athlete's program, because the greater an athlete's maximal strength, the greater their potential for strength endurance. This will improve the amount of force they'll be able to apply for a prolonged period of time. [29] Distance athletes need to have adequate strength endurance to avoid the deterioration of their form as they begin to fatigue. [30] For example, if you're a distance swimmer, it is important that you have the strength to maintain proper form throughout the entire event.

Heavy strength training has also been shown to improve exercise economy in endurance athletes. [31] The term "exercise economy" is used to express the oxygen consumption required to perform a given exercise workload, whether it be spinning, running or any other endurance activity. Moreover, strength imbalances and lack of flexibility are two reasons why endurance athletes get injured. Training to improve overall strength—and increase flexibility—is fundamental to any endurance athlete's resistance training program.

Timing is everything when it comes to incorporating resistance training programs for endurance athletes. Periodization is an organized approach to training that involves progressive cycling of various aspects of a training program during a specific period of time. [32] The best time to begin a resistance training program is in the off season, because in the short term, incorporating resistance training can decrease performance in one's sport. This can come from muscle soreness, as well as having to adapt neuromuscular control due to rapid increases in strength. Honing your endurance sport skills as you adapt to your newfound strength will limit this potential side effect.[33] Periodization is also important to decrease the likelihood of overtraining. Endurance athletes need to find a balance between high-volume training and required rest and recovery.

Here are the top six tips for incorporating resistance training for endurance athletes:

- Taper off (reduce) your resistance training immediately before your endurance event
- Don't start a new resistance training program while "in season"
- Perform your resistance training before your endurance training
- Perform your resistance training on your lighter, lower-intensity days
- Incorporate full-body workouts doing bilateral movements that create symmetry, enhance flexibility, and improve your overall strength

Make sure you're still honing your endurance-sport skills while incorporating a resistance training program.

Key takeaways from this chapter:

- Once you've decided to turn these secrets into lifestyle habits, it's time to create a game plan that's clear and easy to follow.

- You need to develop an action plan so that every time you go into the gym you'll know what you're doing and can focus on intensity and productivity.

- You need to ensure that your program not only meets the demands of your health and fitness goals or sport but, most importantly, is based around having fun and positive reinforcement.

- Timing is everything when it comes to incorporating resistance training programs for endurance athletes.

Chapter 14

The Importance of a Well-Rounded Workout

Whole-body workouts transfer into sports and the rest of your life

Now that the proper nutrients are in your system, they must be utilized. Great news! There's no need to be a slave to the treadmill for hours on end. The secret to efficient exercise is to focus on productivity and leveraging. Productivity is achieving maximum results in minimum time. Leveraging is achieving maximum productivity with minimum effort.

I see way too many teens that have the will but lack the way. For example, many teen boys come into the gym and perform upper body resistance training exercises to make their upper body muscles grow. They spend hours on end every day doing whatever it takes to "get big." Teen girls, on the other hand, tend to shy away from weights and focus their attention on cardiovascular exercise like running, cycling and aerobics. Yet while both of their efforts score an A+, their results are typically a C-. Despite how hard they try, they become overwhelmed with false information that prevents them from seeing real results.

On the teen boy side, most are unaware that if their goal is to get their muscles to grow (muscle hypertrophy), two-thirds of muscle growth is created from the negative. The negative portion of an exercise is when gravity or the cable or machine can do the work for you—when you are controlling the resistance against gravity or lowering the weights. Try mixing in some negative repetitions while training, and more importantly, control the weights during both the negative and positive aspects of the movement, making sure you focus on working the muscles that you're trying to activate.

Moreover, unlike teen girls, most teen boys neglect training their lower body. They feel their legs work enough during cardiovascular exercise and they only care about beach muscles like the chest and arms. However, most teen boys fail to realize that training the lower body is actually the best way to break through a plateau on upper-body muscular growth. Yes, you read correctly—train your legs to grow your arms. But how? Training legs with exercises that focus on large muscle groups—squats, deadlifts and power cleans—releases your body's own anabolic hormones: testosterone, growth hormone (GH) and insulin growth factor 1 (IGF-1). These hormones (specifically GH and IGF-1) play a key role in the repair of muscle tissue, leading to increased body mass. Plus, who wants to have broad shoulders and chicken legs? Having a muscular upper body and skinny little legs is less attractive, and the imbalance can be detrimental when playing a sport.

A muscle-building (hypertrophy) style of resistance training involves a higher volume of training that is progressive in nature. You want to train at a moderate to high intensity of 70-85% of maximum effort with short rest intervals (zero to sixty seconds). Heavy resistance training with short rest intervals builds up more lactic acid and triggers the release of growth hormones. You can increase the production of these muscle-building hormones through training. More frequent stimulation with adequate recovery may produce sustained increases in hormonal responses and the protein synthesis necessary for adding lean muscle mass. Remember, building muscle takes time, and real results are usually not visible until six to eight weeks after beginning a program.

Resistance training is not just for the boys anymore. The weak, subservient girls of the past have been replaced by strong, fit and feminine women. In fashion terms, fit and strong has now replaced skinny as the American ideal. The problem is, many teen girls are afraid that if they lift weights they will get bulky. That just simply isn't the case. First of all, females lack the testosterone levels required to gain the muscle mass that males can gain from resistance training. Men typically have fifteen to twenty times more testosterone than women. Secondly, the reason many teen girls become bulky when lifting weights is that exercise stimulates their appetite and they make poor food choices, like grains and soy, that leave them looking bloated, rather than the right food choices for a fit and feminine physique. The other mistake many teen girls make is resistance training for spot reduction. Spot reduction refers to training a particular muscle group to reduce the body fat over that muscle—for example, doing sit-ups to lose abdominal body fat. The truth is, you cannot spot reduce body fat. If you could, that would mean anyone who eats a lot of food would have a narrow jaw from all that chewing. When designing a resistance-training program for most teen girls, the focus should be on whole body integration. In actuality, both boys and girls would strongly benefit from incorporating whole-body integration into their workout programs.

Think back to one of the most legendary series of movies of all time: *Rocky*. More specifically, go back circa 1985 to *Rocky IV*, where Rocky Balboa comes out of retirement to avenge the loss of Apollo Creed by fighting the super-human Russian named Ivan Drago. On one side, Ivan Drago is shown training for the fight with scientists monitoring his strength and power output on high-tech computers as he does isolated machine-based exercises like the leg press and pec dec fly. On the other side, Rocky Balboa is shown isolated in the middle of the Soviet wilderness, training only with the tools of everyday life. For example, he is shown pulling a wheelbarrow full of bricks, running through knee-high snow, chopping wood with an axe, and shoveling snow. Yet when it came to the fight, all of Rocky's training transferred over to his boxing as he chopped down the Russian to reclaim the heavyweight championship. This style of training and its transfer of conditioning fundamentals into sports and everyday life is one of the main principles behind whole-body integration.

Moreover, triplanar movement training (training within all three planes of motion: sagittal, frontal, and transverse, or front/back, side to side, and rotational) has become a hot topic in progressive fitness training. According to ViPR® fitness equipment creator Michol Dalcourt, it's similar to the complex movement patterns of a working professional like a farmer, a professional mover, or a lumberjack. What we call "working out" they call "chores" or "work." All of the exercises or "chores" that these workers perform involve whole-body integration within multiple planes of motion. For example, when moving a dresser up a set of stairs, a professional mover will lift with their legs and use their upper body muscles to hold and stabilize the load (the dresser) while walking up stairs. Not only are they lifting, but they're also twisting and bending as they move the resistance around tough corners. In a typical gym setting, this would be like doing a step-up while holding a heavy medicine ball in front of you and twisting at the top of the step.

Resistance training will help transform your body into a lean, mean, body-fat-burning machine! For every pound of lean muscle you gain, your body will burn an additional fifty calories per day. By adding a mere three pounds of muscle, your body will burn an additional 150 calories at rest daily. That's roughly equivalent to a thirty-minute walk! This is the reason why bodybuilders can consume vast amounts of calories yet still lose body fat.

When you lift weights, proper mechanics are essential. You're not pushing or pulling a weight from point A to point B. Your muscles are pulling bones through joints in a certain path of motion. Weight training looks easy, but if you don't take proper technique into account, you could injure yourself. You must learn the right way and the wrong way to lift weights so you can spot errors and correct them. This will help you avoid injury, achieve your goals faster, and activate the proper muscles to burn body fat and sculpt that body you've always wanted. Some benefits of weight training include greater muscular strength, improved muscle tone and appearance, increased endurance and enhanced bone density. More importantly, you'll experience a greater level of confidence from the accomplishments you achieve in the gym.

Cardiovascular training makes your internal systems more efficient at utilizing nutrients and helps burn body fat. However, your body adapts to just about any stress you put on it. In order to keep from hitting a plateau, you must change at least one of four variables: frequency (the number of times per week), intensity (how hard you work), modality, (what you are doing) and duration (the length of time). **The most efficient form of cardio for both fat burning and your busy schedule is interval training.** Interval training consists of switching from repetitions of a high-intensity activity to a low to moderate-intensity activity. For example, try sprinting for thirty seconds and then jogging for the next minute. Repeat this series for thirty minutes. You'll burn much more body fat from this type of cardio than simply walking.

Most importantly, increase your daily activity level by finding a sport or an activity that you enjoy. Personally, I prefer to play a sport like basketball, which is physically and mentally stimulating, rather than running or utilizing an indoor cardio machine.

Key takeaways from this chapter:

- You need to develop an action plan so that every time you go into the gym you'll know what you're doing and can focus on intensity and productivity.
- Most teen boys fail to realize that training the lower body is actually the best way to break through a plateau on upper-body muscular growth.

- For both teen boys and girls, resistance training will help transform your body into a lean, mean, body-fat-burning machine!
- Triplanar movement training (training within all three planes of motion: sagittal, frontal, and transverse, or front/back, side to side, and rotational) has become a hot topic in progressive fitness training.

Chapter 15

Rest and Recovery Ensures You Always Bring Your A-Game

When you burn the candle at both ends, everything suffers, including your health and performance

If you were to poll most of the students in your school on the one thing in life they wish they had more of (well, besides money), it would probably be time. Most teens get so busy with multitasking, between school, sports, homework, family and friends, video games, surfing the Internet and cell phones, that in the blink of an eye the day is half over, yet the to-do list still needs to get done.

Because of these obligations and distractions, your sleep suffers. Hey, I can't blame you for wanting to spend an extra hour hanging out with friends, watching an exciting TV show or surfing the web rather than wasting time sleeping. And there's the age-old adage: "You can sleep when you're dead!"

But what if that lost hour or two of sleep each night was responsible for your low energy levels, reduced mental clarity, diminished strength and stamina, inability to grow muscle, and failure to lose body fat? What if not getting enough sleep was keeping you from living a healthy, fit, and successful life? The National Sleep Foundation maintains that school-age kids need 10 to 12 hours of sleep a night and teenagers need between eight and a half and nine and a half hours. Getting sufficient amounts of sleep benefits alertness, memory, problem solving, recovery and muscle building, and overall health. Moreover, most of our poorest nutritional decision-making happens during hours we shouldn't even be awake. A UCSD psychiatry study of more than one million adults found that people who reported sleeping six or more hours each night lived the longest. So maybe the adage should be modified to "You'll die sooner if you don't sleep more."

Like healthy eating and exercise, getting enough quality sleep is fundamental to living a healthy and fit lifestyle. Male lions have it figured out, as they sleep up to twenty hours a day! Bodybuilders are in on the secret, too. **They know that muscle growth occurs during sleep—not when you're training.** Not only does sleep deprivation limit muscle growth but it also zaps your energy for your next workout. Even if you eat right and work out, not getting enough sleep will eventually make you sick and keep you from performing your best. Most of us know the short-term consequences of sleep deprivation from pulling an all-nighter on a project or tossing and turning all night in an uncomfortable bed. Yet most people are unaware of the long-term consequences of not getting enough quality sleep, and even fewer know how to fall asleep and stay asleep.

Our internal biological clock regulates when we should sleep. Sunlight sets this clock to the twenty-four hour sleep/wake cycle of day and night. Sleep deprivation adds up over time, so an hour less per night is like a full night without sleep by the end of the week. The effects of sleep deprivation can lead to health and performance problems, including difficulty with schoolwork, inconsistent performance, decreased attentiveness, body fat gain, increased insulin levels and Type 2 diabetes, hypertension, irritability, cognitive impairment, memory lapse or loss, impaired immune system, decreased reaction times, anxiety, depression, heart disease and growth suppression. Bottom line: when you burn the candle at both ends, everything suffers, and that includes your health and performance.

Instead of sleeping, many teens reach for sodas, energy drinks or coffee for their morning caffeine fix and continually come back throughout the day for more liquid energy. That constant caffeine buzz puts stress on your adrenal glands, which can have negative consequences on both your health and your weight. **By making yourself go to bed a little earlier and ensuring that you get quality sleep, you'll have increased strength and stamina for your workouts, as well as a more efficient and productive day at school thanks to your newfound mental clarity.** All this will leave you with more time at the end of the day and an overall improved quality of life.

So what can you do to ensure you get enough quality sleep? First, exercise will help you sleep better by reducing your stress and anxiety levels. Next, what you put in your body can affect your ability to sleep. Try to minimize or eliminate caffeine completely from your diet. Also, don't work on projects, read, or watch anything stimulating on the television right before you go to bed. This will prevent your mind from racing. Lastly, eliminate all light in your bedroom. A perfect room should be pitch black. This includes your television, your alarm clock (turn it face down or backwards after it's set), and any light from the outside. Light exposure disrupts your circadian rhythm and stimulates the pineal gland in your brain, which reduces your body's ability to produce melatonin and therefore keeps you awake.

OVERTRAINING

Want a sculpted physique or bigger and stronger muscles? *Don't overtrain!* Overtraining is a physical, behavioral, and emotional condition that occurs when the quantity and intensity of an individual's exercise exceeds their recovery capacity. At this point, progress comes to a screeching halt and you start to lose strength and overall fitness. Overtraining is a common problem for weight lifters, but other athletes including runners and swimmers experience it as well. **The moral of the story: it's better to train smart then it is to train too hard.** Remember, training breaks down muscles and proper nutrition and rest and recovery build them back up bigger and stronger than before. Your body needs adequate time to recuperate and regenerate between training sessions. If you continue to exercise at an extreme level without adequate rest, your performance will eventually plateau and then begin to decline. Several days' rest can bring you back from mild overtraining. However, if you push yourself too hard for too long without adequate recovery, it could take weeks or even months to rebound.

So how do you know if you're overtraining? You'll begin to experience symptoms without relief in the form of persistent fatigue, extreme muscle soreness (delayed onset muscle soreness), increased amount of injuries, elevated heart rate, irritability, depression, and even mental breakdown. You may also notice a decrease in strength and an inability to complete your workouts. Lastly, you may feel like your inner drive or enthusiasm for fitness has gone.

What should you do if you hit that wall and are suffering from the symptoms of overtraining? The answer is simple in theory but hard in application. You need to allow more time for your body to recover. You should start by taking some time off from exercise and allow your body to rest and recuperate. Try taking a thirty-to-forty five minute nap during the day for a little recharge. Then, after some time off, reduce your exercise frequency and intensity. Make sure your new program has muscle groups split so that different muscles work on different days. Also make sure that you're eating enough quality food, drinking enough water, and taking enough supplements to handle your training.

Key takeaways from this chapter:

- That lost hour or two of sleep each night is responsible for your low energy levels, reduced mental clarity, diminished strength and stamina, inability to grow muscle, and failure to lose body fat.
- The National Sleep Foundation maintains that school-age kids need ten to twelve hours of sleep a night and teenagers need between eight and a half and nine and a half hours.
- Want bigger and stronger muscles? *Don't overtrain!* Overtraining is a physical, behavioral, and emotional condition that occurs when the quantity and intensity of an individual's exercise exceeds their recovery capacity.

PART 2:

Heart & Mind

of a Champion

Chapter 16

The Character of a Champion

A true champion is a leader both on and off the field

A true champion is a leader in all aspects of life. They focus their efforts not only on making themselves better physically, mentally and emotionally, but on bettering those in their community as well. For instance, a big part of what made Michael Jordan arguably the best athlete of all time was his ability to make everyone around him feel like a winner and believe they could achieve their dreams of being champions.

The responsibility of a true champion is to be a role model in every facet of life—not only in your actions, but how you respond to the actions of others. For example, you may work hard in school and get good grades, treat your family and friends really well, but how do you respond to a social crisis, like bullying, when it's happening around you? Do you stand up for the underdog, or do you turn a blind eye and think to yourself, "That's not my problem"?

So what exactly is bullying? Bullying is an intentional act. It's no accident. **A kid who bullies wants to physically or psychologically harm their victim.** Bullying involves repeated occurrences. It's not generally considered a random act or a single incident. Bullying is when someone is repeatedly picked on or is the constant target of harassment. It's the repeated nature of bullying that causes anxiety and apprehension in victims, such that the anticipation of bullying becomes as problematic as the bullying itself.

Bullying happens when there's a power difference. It's an unfair fight where the bully has some advantage or power over the kid s/he is victimizing. Bullying is not "playing around;" it's about the abuse of power.

Bullying is also an outcome of a group behavior—it's not an individual behavior. When in a group, individual thought disappears and is replaced with what is referred to as "groupthink." It's so utterly human to want to fit in and belong to a group of friends. It's a good thing to have a group of friends with a very strong bond. But the flip side of having an in-group is creating an out-group. **While it's healthy to form strong, bonded groups of friends, you need to be accepting of others and not fight with or victimize the members of the out-group.** This can be a negative consequence of bonding as a group.

When you're a teen, you're searching for an identity. Typically, you find a clique that dresses the same, acts the same, has similar beliefs and values, and listens to the same music. You become part of a group identity and begin to feel comfortable as you develop a sense of belonging. Everyone goes through this process. When I was a kid, I had a falling out with one of my friends my freshman year of high school over a girl I liked that he started dating. I was so upset about it that I needed to get away from my group of friends completely—I just couldn't stand to see the two of them together. So I decided to find a new group of friends.

Fortunately, I was able to step back and realize how many different cliques and groups of people there really were in my high school. Most of my friends were freshmen like me and athletes who listened to popular music and alternative rock. I felt completely lost for about a month. Then, I befriended a sophomore who invited me over to his house and brought me into his group of friends. I was quickly immersed into a new group that had a completely different style— from the clothing they wore to the music they enjoyed to their interest in mischief and partying. Not only did my social life change, but my outlook on life began to mimic those of my new friends. I wish I would have been more true to myself and not felt like I had to change my interests to fit in; but peer pressure is a difficult thing to overcome—and groupthink replaced my individual, rational thought process of what I knew was right and wrong.

People typically address the bullying issue as the behavior of one individual: one student verbally or physically abuses another student. In many cases, the victim's cries for help are ignored. When parents, teachers, or other adults get involved, they typically punish the bully in an attempt to solve the problem. However, the truth is that the bullies don't feel good about themselves. They lack self-esteem and are often victims of some kind of abuse as well. Many times, their actions are learned behaviors from an unstable home or simply a cry for help. Bullies are aggressive and their behavior tends to escalate over time until someone intervenes. Yet while they are bullies in school, many times they are the victims at home. Be open-minded to the idea that these bullies are bullies for a reason. We absolutely need to protect those who are being bullied. However, rather than simply pointing a finger at the bullies and punishing them for their actions, they may need a helping hand to guide them down the right path.

Are you a bully? Before you shake your head "No" and skip over this part of the book, realize that at some point in our lives most of us are bullies and don't even realize it! For example, there are many different types of bullies. We all know if you physically or verbally attack another teenager without reason that you're being a bully. However, people that stand around and watch bullying take place without taking action—let alone laugh as they watch their peers being victimized—can be just as guilty as those who commit the bullying acts themselves.

Imagine there's a kid in your school who simply doesn't fit in. We'll call him Shy Shawn. Shy Shawn just moved to your school from out of state. His clothes are a little different, he talks with a weird accent, he's overweight, and his haircut is kind of funny-looking. Shy Shawn doesn't have any friends and hasn't really bonded with one particular group of people. He doesn't fit in with the choir or drama kids, he's not part of student council, he's not really emo or goth, and he doesn't play a school sport. No one knows much about Shy Shawn, as he's basically a lone wolf and kind of keeps to himself.

Let's take a look at the different types of bullies who are guilty of not helping out our victim, Shy Shawn.

- **Physical Phil**

   Physical Phil is an obvious bully. He's bigger than many of the kids in school and is a bit of a rebel. In order to get a laugh out of his friends and to keep his reputation as one of the stronger and more powerful kids in school, Physical Phil likes to push Shy Shawn around. He bumps him at his locker, throws spitballs in his hair, and has a reputation for pushing around anyone he sees as weak or lame. Physical Phil also raises his hand as if he's going to punch Shy Shawn just to watch him cower.

- **Verbal Valerie**

   Verbal Valerie has a really sharp tongue and likes to pick on Shy Shawn. She says things like, "You have such a big nose. Ewww!" or, "Hey Shawn, it must suck to be so fat. How do you even sit in a chair?" Or, "I have never seen someone so bad at dribbling a basketball." Verbal Valerie builds herself up by talking down to Shy Shawn.

- **Joking Josh**

   Joking Josh likes to mimic Shy Shawn's actions in a way that makes Shy Shawn look dumb. He also cracks jokes around his friends at Shy Shawn's expense. He says things like, "Nice clothes, Shawn. Where did you get them, the dumpster?" He's the one who came up with the name Shy Shawn in the first place. He doesn't consider himself a bully at all because he always hides behind the excuse that he's just joking around and having fun.

- **Laughing Larry**

Laughing Larry is best friends with Physical Phil and Joking Josh. Laughing Larry never physically picks on Shy Shawn or says anything bad to him, but he's always there when Physical Phil is pushing Shy Shawn around or Joking Josh is cracking a joke at Shy Shawn's expense. Laughing Larry is the audience. While he feels like he never does anything wrong and defends himself with, "But I didn't do or say anything!" Laughing Larry has no idea how much his laughter affects Shy Shawn and validates Physical Phil and Joking Josh's poor behavior.

- **Chatty Cathy**

Chatty Cathy never says anything bad to Shy Shawn's face but always gossips about him and spreads rumors. She's like gasoline to a bonfire in that she loves to tell stories behind Shy Shawn's back. She tells her friends things like, "Shy Shawn is such a nerd! Did you hear what he said in biology class today?" Chatty Cathy also posts things on Facebook for all of her friends to see about Shy Shawn—like how he has a gap between his teeth so big that you could drive a semi through it. Chatty Cathy doesn't consider herself a bully whatsoever, as she never says anything bad to Shy Shawn's face. But she wouldn't be caught dead having lunch with Shy Shawn, as he's such a weirdo.

- **Apathetic Annie**

   Apathetic Annie sees how poorly Shy Shawn is being treated by everyone but does nothing about it. While she doesn't agree with what the other kids are doing, she doesn't want to be confrontational with her friends or considered a nark for telling the teachers. Besides, she doesn't even really know Shy Shawn, so why is it her responsibility? This is the reaction of the majority of students.

All of these teens are bullies. If you physically or emotionally attack someone, you are obviously being a bully. Yet if you condone a bully's actions—either by laughing along, joining in, or simply observing their poor actions and not letting an adult know what's going on—you're just as much of a bully as Physical Phil.

What you need to realize is that both bullies and victims want the same things: friendship, acceptance, love, safety and happiness—and bottom line, they both simply want to belong.

Victims like Shy Shawn may eventually forgive you for bullying them as a child, but they'll never forget. Until the day they die, victims will remember these instances and it will shape who they become. It may make them a stronger person or a well-rounded person in the future, but it might also cause them to do something drastic like commit suicide.

Each year, kids like Shy Shawn take their own life to escape the pains of bullying. What might start as a joke could begin to wear Shy Shawn down to the point that he just can't take it anymore. Teens like Shy Shawn will eventually begin to feel like something is wrong with them. They'll feel afraid, sad, mad, embarrassed, empty, alone, frustrated, ashamed, and like they want to disappear. Shy Shawn might even fight back, become a bully himself—or he might just give up on life because he can't take the harassment anymore. Just think—how much would it affect the rest of your life if Shy Shawn committed suicide? What if you jokingly poked fun at Shy Shawn for being different or saw him being bullied and did nothing to stop it? How would you feel?

When I was a kid, I had some of the characteristics of Shy Shawn. In seventh grade, I moved back from San Diego to the small town outside of Chicago where I was born. Throughout junior high and high school, I felt like I was an outsider looking in because I was the only Jewish kid in my class in a town that was predominantly white Anglo-Saxon Protestant. On top of that, I was very shy and sensitive, which many people viewed as angry, and my guarded approach came off as conceited. While I didn't experience much physical bullying, I experienced all of the other types of bullying, even by people I considered to be friends. I felt like I wasn't viewed as Kyle growing up, but more as "Kyle the Jewish kid." I didn't date at all because I was shy and I didn't think parents would want their daughter dating someone who was different. Why did I have to be different? Why couldn't I just be like everyone else? When Christmas came around, I really felt like an outcast. I used to wonder if something was wrong with me because I didn't celebrate Christmas. I felt embarrassed, and every I year counted the days between Christmas and New Year's so I could go back to just being Kyle.

Most of the bullying I experienced was from teens like Joking Josh, Laughing Larry, Chatty Cathy, and Apathetic Annie. And my experiences were a testament to how bullying is truly groupthink. For example, when I would talk to someone one-on-one, they would be nice to me and never say anything demeaning. Yet when I was in a group setting, I would become the butt of all jokes. Kids would constantly poke fun at me for all different reasons, but much of the anti-Semitism I experienced was by walking into conversations or overhearing other people telling Jewish jokes or saying anti-Jewish statements like, "Stop being such a Jew," or, "He Jewed me down." The worst part was when kids wouldn't know that I was Jewish and would repeat very hurtful Jewish Holocaust jokes in front of me. Those instances would push me past my breaking point and lead to me standing up for myself.

Much of the bullying I experienced wasn't because of being Jewish but because I'm non-confrontational by nature and couldn't defend myself. Whenever I did get upset and lose my cool, it made the kids laugh even more knowing they were able to push my buttons. Over time, it began to take its toll on me. There were a couple times in junior high when I became suicidal and considered taking my own life. I never let my parents in on this, but I felt like I was such an outcast. Even though I always had friends, I never felt like I truly fit in or had much to be grateful for in life. I hated everything about the town I lived in, and always feeling like an outsider almost got the best of me. I spent much of my high school years high on marijuana—self-medicating to mask the pain and depression that came with feeling left out. I didn't really have a good grasp on my reasons for living, nor did I have the foresight to know that eventually I would be able to move away and become the person I have become today.

Luckily for me, I was too much of a scaredy cat to actually follow through with my suicidal thoughts, because toward the end of my senior year in high school, I saw the light at the end of the tunnel—I was going to get a fresh start on life in a new town called Bloomington at Indiana University. I decided to invoke the secrets of a champion. I began lifting weights and exercising hard core daily. I changed from a diet of processed junk food and soft drinks to eating healthy, natural foods. I started working on my social skills and coming out of my shy, angry shell. My brother and sister-in-law gave me a fantastic book on the art of flirting that taught me that flirting is not just about hitting on girls—it's about complimenting people and making them feel good about themselves. I studied the traits of the most admired and powerful people in the world and learned that they all have confidence without being arrogant, are empathetic listeners who care for other people, they smile most of the time, they have a passion for helping people, and they have an internal fortitude or inner drive to make the best of any situation.

I have been fortunate to turn my passions into a successful career while building my own healthy, loving and nurturing family. I love my life and now realize that true happiness comes from within, and that if you discover your passions and make them your life's mission, you'll be excited to wake up every morning and live each day to the fullest.

So how do you combat bullying? It's really quite simple. The first thing you do is learn to be more empathetic. Empathy is the ability to understand and share another person's feelings. The first step to becoming empathetic is communication. You don't need to become best friends with Shy Shawn. However, simply walking up to him and offering a compliment like, "Hey Shawn, great job in class today" can significantly alter Shawn's life in ways you may never fully understand. A little bit can go a long way. And as you begin getting to know the real Shawn, rather than just Shy Shawn, you may learn that he has something incredible about him—like he's an amazing guitarist or a fantastic artist. Maybe you and Shawn aren't so different after all. Maybe Shawn will end up owning a successful company in the future and because of your compassion he will be able to help you find a job.

You can't stand up to bullying as an individual. Simply telling a bully what s/he is doing is wrong is only part of the equation. That approach may be too difficult and you may fear that you'll become an outcast like Shy Shawn or that you might be physically or verbally bullied yourself. It takes a group to stand up to a bully. And you now have the power to invoke a serious change in your school, and even within the world. Change starts small and can grow into something really big. It just takes one person to either tell a bully what they are doing is not right or to let an adult, teacher, or coach know what is going on privately so that kids like Shy Shawn can reach their true potential.

Chapter 17

Civic Responsibility of a Champion

A true champion leads a life of self-worth and leaves behind a better legacy

Your generation has grown up dealing with atrocities on American soil from both nature and man that previous generations have not faced. From devastating natural disasters including hurricanes, tornados and earthquakes to atrocities like September 11th, Americans are not used to dealing with so much adversity. The positive effect that has come from these atrocities is a unified sense of community and a desire to give back. For example, according to a 2005 survey by the Higher Education Research Institute at UCLA's Graduate School of Education and Information Studies, 66.3% of incoming college students said it's essential or very important to help others who are in difficulty, the highest response in twenty years. A record 83.2% of incoming college students said they had volunteered at least occasionally during their high school senior year, and 67.3% said there's a good chance they will continue to volunteer in college, also an all-time high. [36]

Yet in this day and age, it's very easy for people to feel like they just don't have enough time in their busy schedules to volunteer. Others simply have no idea how to help. However, there's a new movement rising called "active citizenship." It's the philosophy that as a citizen you can give back by combining your talents and your passions, enabling you to make a substantial impact by helping others.

One of the most satisfying and rewarding experiences you can ever have is to give back. Volunteering involves giving of yourself and your time for a cause without compensation. Volunteering for a noble cause is both a highly rewarding experience and a highly sought-after feature on a young person's resume. Find a charity that's close to your heart and spend some time giving back. Everything that you put into volunteering will be returned to you tenfold.

Now that you've learned the secrets to becoming your best you and begun applying them in your life, you have both the ability and responsibility to use these secrets to help others. The time to act is now. By living the life of a champion and taking just one person who is less fortunate than you under your wing, you can take a significant step toward making the world a better place. A little help goes a long way. And remember from the Character of a Champion chapter: just like when dealing with issues of bullying, the key to combating the crises that are plaguing today's youth is empathy. Empathy is the ability to understand and share another person's feelings. The first step to becoming empathetic is communication. Listen and communicate with others in your community who need your help and then give back by combining your talents and your passions. Start small by asking people how they're doing and listening to their answer. Offer an empathetic ear or lend a hand. You can make a powerful impact by just listening to and helping one person improve their quality of life.

Chapter 18

What Oprah Can't Buy

How time management, will power, and a positive mental attitude will make you richer than a billionaire

Oprah Winfrey is one of the most successful and wealthiest women in the world. While she has done so much for the betterment of society and devoted much of her life to giving back, she has the world at her fingertips. She can afford nearly any material object on the planet and has a staff of people to organize her day and make her life as efficient as possible. While Oprah is a role model on so many levels, her struggle with her weight can teach us all a very valuable lesson: no matter how much money and fame you have, you can't buy health.

If money can't buy health, then what can? The answer is time, will power, and a positive mindset. Do you want to be a multimillionaire or even a billionaire? What's the secret to being even wealthier than a billionaire? The secret to ultimate wealth is your health; and the best news is, for the most part in this game, we start off as equals.

TIME MANAGEMENT

We all have the same amount of time in a day: 24 hours. No one can buy more time. While many people give the excuse that they just don't have enough time to exercise or eat healthy, the facts prove otherwise. According to the Kaiser Family Foundation, the average American youth ages 8 to 18 spends nearly 4 hours a day watching

TV, and almost 2 additional hours on the computer (outside of schoolwork) playing video games. If just one hour of your day was dedicated to physical activity, you'd transform the way you look and feel. The key is time management and making your health a priority. By investing your free time in yourself, you'll earn even more time. For example, by eating right, thinking right, and exercising, your energy levels and mental focus will improve dramatically. This will enable you to breeze through your homework and other responsibilities in less time. You'll earn back even more free time for fun and games.

One of the biggest secrets behind time management is stress management. Most adults don't respect the fact that kids nowadays are under a lot of stress. You have to juggle your overbooked life of school, homework, multiple sports and other after-school activities, family time and fun time. Plus, the competition nowadays in both school and sports is intense!

Stress can leave you overwhelmed and disorganized and sabotage your time management. You can spend more time worrying about everything you have to do and talking about how to do it than actually getting it all done.

Here's a tip: try spending three minutes each day in mindful meditation. Many kids are confused about what meditation really means, and think it involves a lot of work. All mindful meditation means is simply taking a little time out of your day to sit in a quiet place and clear your head so you can refocus your thoughts. While you meditate, try this basic relaxation breathing exercise from Dr. Andrew Weil:

1. Exhale completely through your mouth, making a whoosh sound.
2. Close your mouth and inhale quietly through your nose to a mental count of four.
3. Hold your breath for a count of seven.
4. Exhale completely through your mouth, making a whoosh sound to a count of eight.

This is one breath. Now inhale again and repeat the cycle three more times for a total of four breaths. Breathing exercises like this one can help you regain focus and renew your energy.

The latest study, published in *The Proceedings of the National Academy of Sciences*, shows that only a week of practicing mindful meditation can reduce your stress while improving your mood and ability to pay attention. [37] Other studies show people who practice mindful meditation have increased motivation to make lifestyle changes. Bottom line, this little investment can go a long way.

WILL POWER

What's the secret to spending your time wisely? It's will power. Will power is the ability to control yourself or determine your actions. The more will power you possess, the more you can stand up to the challenges that keep you from achieving your dreams.

Why do most people fail to achieve their health and fitness goals? Despite what most people try to tell themselves, time is not the reason. Six hours of television, Internet and video games is way too much. Money is not the reason—anyone can exercise outside or in their home for free with their own body weight. Genetics is not the reason. Your ancestors are not responsible for doing your grocery shopping, nor are they your ride to the gym! It's mostly self-destructive habits, not fat genes, that are being passed on from your family.

Many people see fitness fanatics and use the excuse of "I wish I had the will power and discipline you have to get fit." They feel like will power is something that you're either born with or not—like brown hair or blue eyes.

The secret to will power is a positive mindset. If you change your mindset to focus on the benefits of an activity rather than the sacrifices, will power will come naturally and effortlessly. You won't think about having the will power to avoid fried and processed convenience foods. Instead, you'll be conscious and aware of how real food makes you feel strong and confident and how junk food makes you feel sick, fat and unhappy. You won't think about how hard it is to motivate yourself to work out. Instead, you'll be excited to go play sports or exercise. You'll thrive on how the happy hormones (endorphins) you release by exercising make you feel on top of the world. A positive mindset generates will power.

POSITIVE MINDSET

I've had the good fortune of being able to work with some of the wealthiest and most successful people in the world—from CEOs of Fortune 500 companies to celebrities to professional athletes. I've worked with multimillionaires who have homes all over the world, luxury cars, private jets, and who live the lifestyle of the rich and famous. I also had the privilege of being raised in a blue collar, small Midwestern town where people struggle to make ends meet. Many of the people I grew up with believe that if they only had more money, all of their problems would go away and they'd be happy and healthy. Yet spending my days among the financially elite, I've seen that many wealthy people are equally miserable, as money cannot buy happiness or health. This is because happiness and health cannot be bought. Instead, they need to be built from within you.

It's really not hard to be healthy and active. It's simply making a choice to change the way you see yourself. You need to start visualizing yourself as healthy and active. You become your thoughts. Start by changing how you talk about yourself from "I'm trying to be healthy and active" to "I am healthy and active because it makes me happy."

The same thing goes for the "diet mentality." One of the biggest mistakes most people make is that when they're ready to make a change they proclaim, "I'm going on a diet!" "I'm going to lose (fill in the blank) pounds by (fill in the blank) time." Then they follow it up with a negative comment like "I'm sick of this muffin top of fat on my hips" or "I need to lose this gut. I can't even fit into my pants!" As a personal trainer, I hear these types of comments nearly every day. The first thing I do with these clients is redirect their mindset. A diet is not the solution. What are the first three letters in diet? D-I-E! The pain and suffering mentality of dieting leads the overwhelming majority of people to fail at making health and fitness a part of their lives.

According to Stanford University professor Dr. Carol Dweck, the view you adopt for yourself profoundly impacts the way you lead your life.

"Most kids don't understand the power of their beliefs. These may be beliefs we're aware of or unaware of, but they strongly affect what we want and whether we succeed in getting it. This tradition also shows how changing people's beliefs—even the simplest beliefs—can have profound effects." [38]

A positive mindset is not about fooling yourself into believing that living a healthy lifestyle is easy. It's about believing that it's worth it.

PART 3:

The Game

Plan

Chapter 19

Taking the First Step

How to execute your plan of action and achieve your goals

You have to be hungry for it. You have to want it. You have to be willing to do whatever it takes to get it. But how do you take that first step? The best advice is to take baby steps and keep it fun. This is not an overnight fix or an extreme makeover. Becoming the person you want to be is a journey of trial and error. Remember, setbacks are a normal part of human behavior. Don't fall into the setback mentality that if you fall off the wagon you blew it and aren't allowed back on. A common mistake is to think, "I already had one cookie, so I might as well have ten." But it's much easier to burn off that one cookie than to burn off nine more.

Just like a professional athlete, you need a team of specialists. We at Strive 4 Fitness® are now your team of specialists who will help you improve your quality of life. Applying any of the health secrets in this book to your lifestyle will make a dramatic impact on your fitness, health, and happiness.

Take responsibility and realize that you have complete control over what you put into your body. Your health and appearance are a reflection of your choices. Remember, nobody likes procedures, but everybody loves great results. Following through with this program will take hard work and sacrifice, but the rewards will improve every aspect of your life. And once these lifestyle changes become your habits, you will begin to love the process. Train your mind to enjoy the benefits of a healthy and fit lifestyle, rather than feeling as though you're suffering under self-deprivation. Remember, you need to enjoy the ride.

HABIT

I am your constant companion. I am your greatest helper or heaviest burden. I will push you onward or drag you down to failure. I am completely at your command. Half the things you do you might just as well turn over to me, and I will be able to do them quickly and correctly.

I am easily managed. You must merely be firm with me. Show me exactly how you want something done and after a few lessons I will do it automatically. I am the servant of all great men; and, alas, of all failures as well. Those who are great, I have made great. Those who are failures, I have made failures.

I am not a machine, though I work with all the precision of a machine and the intelligence of a man. You may run me for a profit or run me for ruin—it makes no difference to me.

Take me, train me, be firm with me and I will place the world at your feet. Be easy with me and I will destroy you.

WHO AM I? I AM HABIT!

—Anonymous

Chapter 20

The 21-Day Strive 4 Fitness® Game

Your kick-start to transform the way you look, feel, and think in just 21 days

Appendix 1: Commitment to My Success Contract

I, _____, am committed to taking control of my health and fitness. I promise to give the 21-Day Strive 4 Fitness® Game my best effort. While I know it won't be easy, I'm going to work hard to develop the healthy eating and lifestyle patterns I need to be successful. I understand that I must journal the process until I develop healthy eating and lifestyle patterns or if I begin to plateau.

For 21 days, I will:

- **Think like a champion**
- **Eat like a champion**
- **Play like a champion**
- **Re-energize like a champion**

This will help me learn how best to manage both my health and fitness as I strive to achieve my goals. This will make me a conscious performer instead of an unconscious spectator. I know that failing to plan is planning to fail, and that the habits I develop will benefit me for the rest of my life.

_____   _____
Print Your Name   Print Your Witness's Name

_____   _____

Signature   Signature

_____   _____

Date   Date

Appendix 2: FIT Score Assessment

Informed Consent Disclaimer

All nutritional programs are simply recommendations, not prescribed diets, based on our theories of optimal nutrition and have not been scientifically proven. The following information is for educational and informational use only.

Strive 4 Fitness LLC and Kyle Brown assume no responsibility for the correct or incorrect use of our information. Any information we provide and any recommendations we make should not be used to, nor are they intended to, nor do they in fact diagnose, treat, cure or mitigate any specific health problem. Anyone with any health complaint should seek the care and consultation of an appropriate licensed health practitioner. No attempt should be made to use any information we provide as a form of treatment for any specific condition without the approval and guidance of a physician.

I understand that participating in any program of exercise, nutrition and lifestyle change has certain risks. The information I have supplied is correct to the best of my knowledge. I also acknowledge that all participants in any program should consult their physician before embarking on such a program. I take full responsibility for my participation in any of these programs for any claims for injuries or illness that may result from my participation in any of these programs.

Note: If you are a minor, please have expressed written permission from a parent or guardian before beginning any fitness program.

Important Directions (Please Read):

1. Photocopy this form or write your answers down on a separate piece of paper. You can also print this form off at www.thezebrabook.com. We encourage you to create a profile at www.thezebrabook.com, where you can record your scores online. You will be retesting your "Fit Score" after you complete the 21-Day Strive 4 Fitness® Game, as well as every 21 days until you reach your goals, or if you ever get off track.

2. Answer each question with the answer that best fits your current situation. Don't answer the questions with what you think you should answer, as it will throw off your scores and keep you from making the necessary lifestyle changes to help you achieve your goals.

3. Add up the numbers for each section for your total for that section.

4. Match your scores with the appropriate rating on the FIT Score Chart below.

5. Add all four sections' scores together to figure out your Fit Score.

FIT SCORE PART 1: THINK LIKE A CHAMPION

1. Have you ever had a workout partner?

    a. Yes (5 points)

    b. No (0 points)

2. Have you ever set and reviewed your fitness goals?

    a. Yes (5 points)

    b. No (0 points)

3. Have you ever created a fitness mantra to motivate you to achieve your fitness goals?

    a. Yes (5 points)

    b. No (0 points)

4. When you see someone being picked on, do you:

    a. Step in and stop the kid(s) who are bullying or inform an adult or teacher (5 points)

    b. Join in (0 points)

    c. Laugh (0 points)

    d. Avoid the kid being picked on out of fear of being associated with them (0 points)

5. Do you regularly do your part to help out around the house?

    a. Yes (5 points)

    b. No (0 points)

6. How often do you volunteer your time to help make your community a better place?

    a. Once a month or more (5 points)

    b. Every other month up to once per month (4 points)

    c. Twice per year up to every other month (2 points)

    d. One or fewer times per year (0)

7. After you have a good workout, how often do you congratulate yourself for doing a good job taking care of your health and fitness?

    a. Never (0 points)

    b. Sometimes (3 points)

    c. Always (5 points)

8. When you succeed in something (good grades, helping out in your community, etc.), how often do you congratulate yourself for doing a good job?

    a. Never (0 points)

    b. Sometimes (3 points)

    c. Always (5 points)

9. How often do you worry (i.e. about school, home, friends, or other problems)?

    a. Every day (0)

    b. Every few days (1)

    c.   Once a week (3)

    d.   Rarely if ever (5)

10. How would you rate your overall happiness with the way you look and feel?

    a.   Unhappy, and I don't see any way I am going to make a change for the better (0)

    b.   Fair, and I don't see any way I am going to make a change for the better (0)

    c.   Fair, and I see myself making changes for the better (3)

    d.   I am happy with the way I look and feel (5)

FIT SCORE PART 2: EAT LIKE A CHAMPION

1.   How often do you eat vegetables (not including potatoes or French fries)?

    a.   Less than three times per week (0 points)

    b.   Every other day (1 point)

    c.   Once daily (3 points)

    d.   Two or more times daily (5 points)

2.   Do you eat more raw vegetables than cooked?

    a.   No (0 points)

    b.   Yes (5 points)

3.   How often do you eat white bread, white rice, pasta, or pizza?

   a.   Four or more times per week (0)

   b.   Every other day (3)

   c.   Once a week or less (5)

4.   What do you typically eat for breakfast?

   a.   Nothing (0)

   b.   Muffins or pastries (0)

   c.   Cereal, toast or bagels (0)

   d.   Oatmeal and/or fruit (3)

   e.   Protein shake, eggs, or yogurt (5)

5.   What do you normally eat for snacks?

   a.   Nothing (0)

   b.   Cookies, candy, chips, or other packaged foods (0)

   c.   Fruit, dairy, vegetables, nuts and seeds (5)

6.   How much water do you drink a day?

   a.   None (0)

   b.   One to five eight ounce glasses (2)

   c.   Six to ten eight ounce glasses (3)

    d. More than ten eight ounce glasses (5)

7. What do you typically eat for lunch at school?

    a. Nothing (0)

    b. Pizza, pasta, pastries, or candy (0)

    c. Sandwiches (3)

    d. Salads with protein, or chicken, beef, fish, or vegetables and fruits (5)

8. What do you typically eat for dinner?

    a. Starch (pasta, pizza, bread, rice) (0)

    b. Fast food (0)

    c. Fried protein (chicken, beef, turkey, or fish) (2)

    d. Baked or grilled protein (chicken, beef, turkey, or fish) (5)

9. How often do you eat packaged desserts from stores (cake, candy, ice cream, pies, etc.)?

    a. Daily (0)

    b. Every other day (1)

    c. Three times a week (3)

    d. Two times a week or less (5)

10. How often do you use artificial sweeteners?

    a.   Three or more times per week (0)

    b.   One to three times per week (1)

    c.   Never (5)

11. How often do you eat fast food?

    a.   Three or more times per week (0)

    b.   One to three times per week (3)

    c.   Never or rarely (5)

12. Do you regularly skip meals?

    a.   Yes (0)

    b.   No (5)

13. Do you typically eat high-starch or sugar carbohydrates alone (bread, chips, bagels, cookies, pasta, candy, muffins)?

    a.   Yes (0)

    b.   No (5)

14. How often do you drink caffeinated or high sugar drinks (soda, fruit juice, energy drinks, etc.)?

    a.   Daily (0)

    b.   Every other day (2)

    c.   Occasionally or never (5)

15. How often do you go more than four hours without eating?

    a.   Daily (0)

    b.   Every other day (2)

    c.   Occasionally (3)

    d.   Rarely or never (5)

FIT SCORE PART 3: PLAY LIKE A CHAMPION

Watch the "Play Like a Champion" FIT Score Test Video at www.strive4fitness.com for exercise demonstrations, and follow along, filling in the scorecard as you go. Before you start, do a light warm-up:

    A. Jog in place 30 seconds
    B. Jumping jacks 30 seconds
    C. 30 seconds of squats
    D. 30 seconds of push-ups

Notes: Don't hold your breath, and take a maximum of two minutes' rest between each exercise.

1.   How many quality push-ups (knee or regular) can you do in one minute? (Down 1 second, hold 1 second, up 1 second)

    a.   0-5 (0)

    b.   6-10 (2)

   c.   11-15 (3)

   d.   16-20 (4)

   e.   21+ (5)

2.   How many quality high knees can you do in one minute?
(Note: Count both sides as one repetition)

   a.   0-20 (0)

   b.   21-30 (2)

   c.   31-40 (3)

   d.   41-50 (4)

   e.   51+ (5)

3.   How long can you hold a plank?

   a.   0-20 seconds (0)

   b.   21-30 seconds (2)

   c.   31-50 seconds (3)

   d.   51-60 seconds (4)

   e.   61+ (5)

4.   How many 10 ft. lateral shuffles can you do in one minute?

   a.   0-10 (0)

   b.   11-20 (2)

    c.   21-30 (3)

    d.   31-40 (4)

    e.   41+ (5)

5. How many quality mountain climbers can you do in one minute?

    a.   0-10 (0)

    b.   11-20 (2)

    c.   21-30 (3)

    d.   31-40 (4)

    e.   41+ (5)

6. How many ice skaters can you do in one minute? (Jump on one leg side to side and back, the other foot all the way behind you)

    a.   0-10 (0)

    b.   11-20 (2)

    c.   21-40 (3)

    d.   41-50 (4)

    e.   51+ (5)

7. How many squat jumps can you do in one minute?

  a. 0-10 (0)

  b. 11-20 (2)

  c. 21-30 (3)

  d. 31-40 (4)

  e. 41+ (5)

8. How many Burpees can you do in one minute? (Kick legs out/in then jump, no push-up included)

  a. 0-3 (0)

  b. 4-7 (2)

  c. 8-10 (3)

  d. 11-15 (4)

  e. 16+ (5)

9. How many butt kicks can you do in one minute?

  a. 0-10 (0)

  b. 11-30 (2)

  c. 31-40 (3)

  d. 41-50 (4)

  e. 51+ (5)

EFFORT POINTS:

10. How often do you either play sports (i.e. basketball, soccer, tennis), do cardiovascular exercise (i.e. running, biking, swimming) or resistance training (i.e. weight lifting, bodyweight exercises, gymnastics) or an unorganized, un-coached game or activity (i.e. tag, skateboarding, pick-up ball)?

    a.   Rarely or never (0)

    b.   Once a week (2)

    c.   Two to four times a week (4)

    d.   Five to six times a week (6)

    e.   30 to 60 minutes a day (8)

    f.   At least 60 minutes a day (10)

FIT SCORE PART 4: RE-ENERGIZE LIKE A CHAMPION

1.   How often do you sit in a quiet place or listen to relaxing music and clear your head so you can refocus your thoughts?

    a.   Rarely or never (0)

    b.   Once a week (1)

    c.   Two to four times per week (3)

    d.   Four or more times per week (5)

2.   Do you typically feel tired after lunch?

a. Yes (0)

b. No (5)

3. How often do you typically wake up during the night?

   a. More than twice (0)

   b. One or two times (3)

   c. Rarely or never (5)

4. How many hours of sleep do you get on a typical night?

   a. Five hours or less (0)

   b. Six or seven hours (1)

   c. Seven to eight and a half hours (3)

   d. Eight and a half hours or more (5)

5. How often do you wake up feeling like you need more sleep?

   a. Three or more times per week (0)

   b. One to three times per week (3)

   c. Rarely or never (5)

FIT SCORE RESULTS:

≤ 100: Bronze Medal

101–159: Silver Medal

≥ 160: Gold Medal

Appendix 3: Strive 4 Fitness Game Rules of the Game

*LEAN *FIT *ATHLETIC *STRONG *HAPPY *HEALTHY *ENERGIZED

What if I was to tell you that in just 21 days you can transform the way you live your life? It's true! By taking your health and fitness in your own hands, you're going to look better, feel better, and have more energy. You'll kick start your journey to optimal health and fitness and enjoy the benefits for the rest of your life! Are you ready? Let's do this!

PART #1: THINK LIKE A CHAMPION

1. Team Up!

The first step to success is to find a teammate. A teammate is a friend or a mentor that is ready to make the change with you! If you cannot find someone who will be on the plan, at least find someone to report to who will hold you accountable. This can be a parent, a friend, a teacher, or any role model who will be your partner on your fitness journey. Accountability is key to success as having a fitness buddy will keep you on track and make the whole process more fun.

2. Establish Your Goals

Write down 3 reasons why you want to make this change.
Remember, the universal goal of this game is to improve your quality of life! Fat loss, increased energy, looking better, and feeling

healthier is all by products. Awareness of this goal will keep this a lifestyle rather than a diet.

(Examples: I want to be strong. I want to be a role model for my family. I want to feel more athletic. I want to fit better in my clothes. I want to have more energy. I want to look as good on the outside as I feel on the inside.)

a. _____

b. _____

c. _____

3. Create your new daily fitness mantra

A mantra is a phrase that you constantly repeat to yourself that will help you achieve what you want. Mantras are always said in the present tense. You can create your own or use one or any of the examples listed.

(Examples:

a. "I am doing this for myself. This program works. I will never give up!"
b. "I look good because I take care of myself!"
c. "Every day I get stronger!"
d. "I believe in myself. I believe in this program. This is my time to succeed!")

My new fitness mantra is:

_____

Now write this down on a piece of paper and tape it on a place you will see each day, like your bedroom door, your bathroom mirror, or inside your school binder. **The more you keep focused on your fitness mantra and why you are making these changes, the better chance they become lifestyle habits.**

4. Look Out For Others

A true champion is a leader both on and off the field. They focus their efforts not only on making themselves better physically, mentally and emotionally—but on bettering those around them in their community as well. Every day during the 21-day Strive 4 Fitness® game, challenge yourself to step outside your comfort zone and simply talk to someone at school you don't really know. Not only will you be doing your part to combat the bullying crisis; but also by learning how to be empathetic, you may alter someone's life for the better and even make a new friend.

In this game, you will earn points for being kind to or helping out someone at school you barely know, helping out around your house, and for mentoring someone else playing the game.

5. Acknowledge Your Successes

Every day when you finish your exercise, think about how good you feel. Focus on the energy and power you have after a good workout. Notice how the happy hormones (endorphins) take over your body while your stress disappears. Be proud of this accomplishment and recognize why you need to replicate it tomorrow.

PART #2: EAT LIKE A CHAMPION

This new way of eating will provide you a balance of nutrients to fuel your body for optimal health and performance. You will lose excess body fat, look and feel better, and have more energy!

Be realistic! Most programs will work for some people but will fail for most people. The realistic, healthy and balanced lifestyle program you follow is better than the perfect diet you quit. You don't need to be perfect! You just need to be better today than yesterday. You can still eat deserts. You can still enjoy your favorite foods. A little effort goes a long way. You just need to start by making one change, like eating a protein-packed breakfast, and you'll see amazing results!

<u>**Remember these success tips:**</u>

1. **This is not a diet!** Diets don't work because they are unrealistic in the long-term as they involve unnatural eating patterns that can't be maintained. That is why 98% of Americans who lose weight gain it back, and then some, within 1 year.

2. You have complete control over what you put into your body. If you choose wisely, your health and appearance will become a reflection of this fact.

3. There is nothing better for your health or fat loss than quality water in optimal quantities.

4. You can reeducate your taste buds so that the most nutritious foods become the most delicious foods

5. Replacing processed foods with real whole foods is essential for success.

Now shop for your energizing foods off your grocery list and follow the sample menu as close as possible. Circle the foods you eat and the beverages you drink. You will earn points for your good choices and lose points for your bad choices.

Prepare for setbacks. Stuff happens. Don't let setbacks keep you from moving forward. Just because you have an unhealthy meal or dessert or miss a workout doesn't mean that you should give up! No one expects you to be perfect and you shouldn't put that pressure on yourself.   Also, if you hear negative comments from other kids, friends, or relatives brush it off. They are just jealous that you have a plan and have taken action.

PART #3: PLAY LIKE A CHAMPION

1. Make sure you get at least 60 minutes of play every day. This could be your favorite sport (like basketball or soccer) or cardiovascular exercise like running, biking, or swimming. It could also include weight-bearing exercises in or out of the gym.

2. Try our 30-minute Playground workout. This can be done anywhere and requires no equipment.

3. Have fun! Exercise and working out doesn't have to be work! Discover your fitness passions and find a sport or activity that makes you happy while making you healthy.

PART #4: RE-ENERGIZE LIKE A CHAMPION

1. Sleep yourself healthy

Just like you need to plug in your cell phone or laptop to recharge at the end of the day, your body needs time to rest and recover to heal itself. Without enough quality sleep, your health and fat loss will both be hindered. As a teenager, you need to get between 8 ½ and 9 ½ hours of sleep each night. For every lost hour of sleep, you will lose a point.

2. Mindful Meditation: Take 3 for Me™

Spend three minutes each day in mindful meditation. Many kids are confused about what meditation really means, and think it involves a lot of work. All mindful meditation means is simply taking a little time out of your day to sit in a quiet place or listen to relaxing music and clear your head so you can refocus your thoughts. While you meditate, try this basic relaxation breathing exercise from Dr. Andrew Weil:

a. Exhale completely through your mouth, making a whoosh sound.

b. Close your mouth and inhale quietly through your nose to a mental count of four.

c.   Hold your breath for a count of seven.

d.   Exhale completely through your mouth, making a whoosh sound to a count of eight.

e.   This is one breath. Now inhale again and repeat the cycle three more times for a total of four breaths. Breathing exercises like this one can help you regain focus and renew your energy.

3. Hour To Devour™

While you are making the change to a healthy lifestyle, it's ok to occasionally treat yourself with a less healthy meal or dessert. This will keep you on track and in the game. Enjoy your "Hour to Devour ™ guilt-free 1 to 2 times per week. You deserve it!

Get Excited! You have already started the process of change. You can do this and you're going to love the results! Get psyched that starting today everything is going to change in your favor. Starting today, you are on the path to greatness. The first step to success is to create a mindset of success. It's all connected: nutrition, exercise, and state of mind. Just do your best! Remember, like everything else in life, your hard work will pay off. The more you put into this game, the more you'll succeed!

Appendix 4: Strive 4 Fitness Game Scorecard

Go to www.thezebrabook.com and register online to play the 21-Day Strive 4 Fitness® Game. Here, you can keep track of your score. You can print out copies of the Game Scorecard as well to keep track of your points during the game.

PART 1: THINK

Daily Teammate Check-in = 10 bonus points

Review your goals = 5 points

Say fitness mantra = 5 points

Be kind to or help out someone at school you barely know = 5 points

Mentor someone else playing the game = 5 points

Help out around the house = 5 points

Acknowledge your successes = 5 points

Read a chapter of *How Much Does A Zebra Weigh?*, watch one of our nutrition or exercise videos, or read a fitness article = 5 points (max 5 points)

_____ TOTAL

MEDALS:

40 points or more = Gold

30 to 40 points = Silver

20 to 30 points = Bronze

< 20 points = No medal

PART 2: EAT

PROTEIN

(Note: Eat 2-4 servings per meal depending on your size, amount of lean muscle mass, amount of physical activity, and fitness goals.)

<u>Options:</u>

Each ounce of beef, poultry, or fish = 1 point (max 10 points)

____ points

Each egg = 1 point (max 3 points)

____ points

Each serving of dairy = 1 point (max 1 point)

____ point

Each serving FIT 365® = 3 points (max 6 points)

____ points

Each serving Perfect Foods bars = 2 points (max 2 points)

____ points

CARBOHYDRATES

Options:

Fruit

(Note: Eat 1-3 servings a day. Keep limited or eliminate if you have cancer, diabetes, or hypoglycemia.)

Each piece of fruit = 1 point (max 3 points)

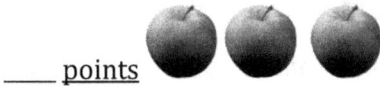

___ points

Vegetables

(Note: Eat minimum 4-8 servings/day within 2-3 meals. Veggies should make up half of your plate.)

Each serving of vegetables = 2 points (max 10 points)

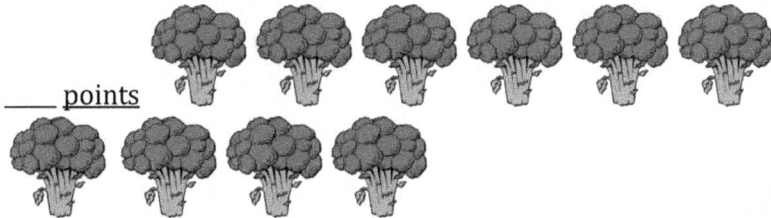

___ points

STARCH

(Note: Eat 0-2 servings per day. Keep as limited as possible if you have body fat loss goals and for optimal health.)

Starch: 2 servings per day limit = 0 points. Anything over 2 servings = -2 points

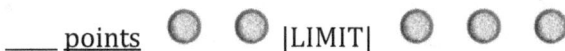

___ points |LIMIT|

HEALTHY FATS AND OILS

(Note: Eat roughly 2-5 servings per day depending on your size, amount of lean muscle mass, amount of physical activity, fitness goals, and the fat content of your protein sources. For example, eating higher fat protein sources like beef or salmon will require fewer fat servings throughout the day.)

<u>Options:</u>

Each serving of nuts and seeds = 1 point (max 3 points)

____ <u>points</u> |LIMIT|

Each serving healthy oils = 1 point (max 3 points)

____ <u>points</u> |LIMIT|

Each serving of non-dairy milk substitutes = 1 point (max 2 points)

____ <u>points</u> |LIMIT|

BEVERAGES

(Note: Goal is 1 oz. per pound bodyweight)

Each 8 fl. oz. glass of water = 1 point (max 10 points)

____ <u>points</u>

Each cup of tea = 0 points (2 cups max)

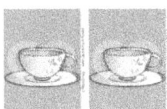

-____ points |LIMIT|

Each 8 fl. oz. soda = -3 points

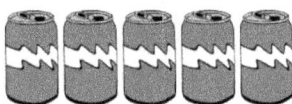

-____ points

Each processed, packaged food = -3 points

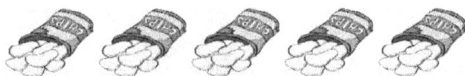

-____ points

Each serving sweets or desserts = -3 points

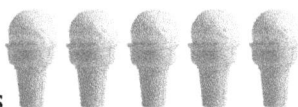

-____ points

_____ TOTAL SCORE

MEDALS:

30 points or more = Gold

20 to 30 points = Silver

10 to 20 points = Bronze

< 10 points = No Medal

PART 3: PLAY

_____ Minutes Sports

_____ Minutes Cardio

_____ Minutes Resistance

_____ TOTAL =   +   +

MEDALS:

60 minutes or more = Gold

30 to 59 minutes = Silver

10 to 29 minutes = Bronze

< 10 minutes = No medal

PART 4: RE-ENERGIZE

Sleep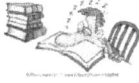

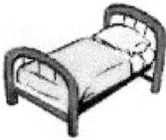 _____ hours

1 point per hour of sleep

_____ points

Take 3 For Me = 5 points (max 5 points)

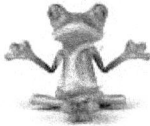

_____ points

Enjoy 1-2 Hour to Devour™ meals guilt-free per week = 5 points (max 10 points per week)

_____ points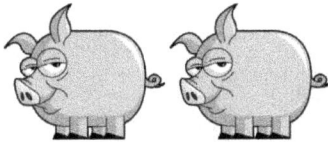

_____ TOTAL SCORE

MEDALS:

21 points or more = Gold

15 to 20 points = Silver

11 to 14 points = Bronze

< 10 points = No medal

MEDALS:

GOLD

You are achieving your potential and ready to live the life of a champion!

SILVER

You are on your way to living a healthy lifestyle! You've made some great improvements and are ready to strive for the gold.

BRONZE

You are making some changes, but you deserve better! Time to take it to the next level and earn that silver medal!

Appendix 5: Grocery Shopping Made Easy

Key Points:

1. Choose organic vegetables and fruits when possible—
    especially the ones where you eat the skin.

2. When possible, avoid packaged and processed foods that are
    full of preservatives and additives. Stick mostly to the
    outside aisles of the grocery store, where they sell fresh, real
    food, rather than the middle rows where you'll find packaged
    foods.

3. Try one new option in each category every week. Place an "X"
    to the left of the grocery item you want to try. Your goal is to
    learn to enjoy a variety of foods as you fight food boredom.

PROTEIN SOURCES:

MEATS

Best Options	Other Options
Beef (< 20% fat)	Lean Pork
Buffalo/Bison (ground or burger patties)	
Lamb	
Goat	
Venison	
Elk	

*   Choose grass-fed, organic meats when possible

POULTRY & EGGS

Chicken
Chicken Eggs
Turkey
Duck
Ostrich
Pheasant
Quail
Cornish Game Hen

* Choose organic, free-range, hormone-free and antibiotic-free poultry when possible

FISH AND OTHER SEAFOOD

Best Options	Other Options
Salmon	Crab
Halibut	Lobster
Cod	Clams
Tilapia	Rockfish
Tuna	Shrimp
Mahi-Mahi	Crayfish
Orange Roughy	Whitefish
Sea Bass	Sardines

	Red Snapper	Scallops
		Shrimp
		Squid
		Catfish
		Grouper
		Trout
		Herring
		Mackerel
		Perch
		Arctic Char

*   Choose wild, cold-water fish whenever possible

CARBOHYDRATE SOURCES:

VEGETABLES

Artichoke	Okra
Arugula	Olives (all types)
Asparagus	Peppers (Bell; all colors)
Bamboo Shoots	Peppers (Hot; all colors)
Beets	Pumpkin
Bok Choy	Radishes
Broccoli	Red Leaf Lettuce
Brussels Sprouts	Red Potatoes

Cabbage	Romaine Lettuce
Carrots	Scallions
Cauliflower	Shallots
Celery	Spinach
Collard Greens	Sprouts
Cucumber	Sweet Potatoes
Eggplant	Tomatoes
Green Beans	Turnips
Leeks	Watercress
Mushrooms	Water Chestnut
Mustard Greens	Yams
Onions	Zucchini

* Choose pesticide-free options when possible

SEA VEGETABLES

Agar	Kelp
Arame	Kombu
Dulce	Nori
Hijiki	Wakame

FRUITS

Apples	Kiwi
Apricots	Lemons
Bananas	Limes
Blackberries	Mangos
Blueberries	Nectarines
Boysenberries	Papayas
Cantaloupe	Passion Fruit
Casaba Melon	Peaches
Cherries	Persimmon
Coconut	Plums
Cranberries	Dried Plums
Dates	Pineapple
Elderberries	Pomegranate
Grapefruit (pink or red)	Raspberries
Grapes	Rhubarb
Guava	Strawberries
Honeydew Melon	Watermelon

* Choose pesticide-free options when possible.

STARCH (CARBOHYDRATE) SOURCES:

BREADS, CEREALS, TORTILLAS, GRAINS, AND PASTAS

Whole Grain Options	Ready-Made Food Options
Brown Rice	Couscous
Corn	Corn Tortillas
Oatmeal (steel cut if possible)	Sprouted Breads (i.e. Ezekiel Bread)
Quinoa	Whole Grain Bagels
Spelt	Whole Grain Bagels
Whole Wheat (sprouted)	Whole Grain Pastas
Wild Rice	Whole Wheat Breads

- Choose any of the above whole grain options for each ready-made food type
- Choose gluten-free options when possible

BEANS AND OTHER LEGUMES

Black Beans	
Garbanzo Beans	
Lentils	
Navy Beans	
Pinto Beans	

- Count as a starch source, not a protein source
- For vegetarians, mix rice and beans or eat quinoa or spirulina for complete protein sources.

HEALTHY FAT SOURCES

NUTS AND SEEDS

Almonds		Roasted Peanuts
Brazil Nuts		Pecans
Cashews		Pine Nuts
Chia Seeds		Pistachios
Roasted Chestnuts		Poppy Seeds
Filberts		Pumpkin Seeds
Ground Flax Seeds		Sesame Seeds
Hazelnuts		Sunflower Seeds
Hickory Nuts		Walnuts
Macadamia Nuts		

* Choose raw, unsalted options when possible.

HEALTHY OILS

Virgin Coconut Oil
Extra Virgin Olive Oil
Fish Oil/Cod Liver Oil
Flaxseed Oil

DAIRY

Blue Cheese		Greek Yogurt
Brie		Kefir
Butter		Monterey Jack
Buttermilk		Mozzarella
Cheddar		Muenster
Colby		Neufchatel
Cottage Cheese		Parmesan
Cow's Milk		Provolone
Cream		Raw Milk
Cream Cheese		Ricotta
Feta		Romano
Ghee		Swiss
Goat Cheese		Sour Cream
Goat Milk		Yogurt (organic, no sugar added)
Gouda		

- Choose raw, unpasteurized dairy when possible
- Choose yogurt as a protein source and cheese as a healthy fat source

NON-DAIRY MILK OPTIONS

Almond Milk (low calorie vanilla or chocolate, or original flavors)
Coconut Milk (low calorie vanilla or chocolate, or original flavors)
Hemp Milk (low calorie vanilla or chocolate, or original flavors)

HEALTHY MEAL AND SNACK REPLACEMENT SHAKES, BARS, AND SUPPLEMENTS

B & C Vitamin Packets	Greens Power
Coconut Oil	Multi-vitamin Multi-mineral
Coconut Water	Perfect Foods® bars
Glutamine	Probiotics
Fish Oil or Krill Oil	Psyllium Seed Husk Fiber
FIT 365® Chocolate and Vanilla Complete Nutritional Shakes	
Ground Flaxseed	
Flaxseed Oil	

CONDIMENTS

Organic BBQ Sauce
Organic Ketchup
Honey
Hot Sauce
Mustard
Organic Pasta Sauce
Fresh Salsa

HERBS & SPICES

Basil	Ginger
Black Pepper	Herb Teas
Cayenne Pepper	Parsley
Cilantro	Oregano
Cinnamon	Sea Salt
Cumin	Stevia (sweetener)
Garlic	Green, Red, White, Black Teas

Appendix 6: Sample Daily Menu

Conscious Eating 101:

1. Slow down and savor your food! Chew each bite thoroughly and allow time for your body to tell you when it's content. You'll end up eating less and only what your body really needs.
2. Eat until you're satisfied, not stuffed and bloated.
3. Drink primarily water instead of soda, sugar drinks, and artificial juices.
4. Adjust your portion sizes up or down based on whether you're an elementary school, middle school, or high school boy or girl. Stay between the portion guidelines in the sample menu when possible.
5. Enjoy your Hour to Devour™ one to two times per week! This is where you can include desserts.

BREAKFAST	A.M. SNACK	SCHOOL LUNCH	P.M. SNACK	DINNER
Option #1: 2 boiled or scrambled eggs (see *Quick Scrambler* recipe) 1 cup berries 1 slice sprouted toast	Option #1: organic yogurt apple, pear, or peach Option #2: Perfect Foods bar mini Option #3: raw	Option #1: sliced turkey sprouted tortilla or bread 1 cup of tomatoes, peppers, onions, and lettuce mustard	Any power snack recipe	Option #1: Any satisfying salad recipe Option #2: Any amazing protein dish recipe with any side dish

Option #2:	almonds	¼ avocado		recipe
2 scoops FIT 365 chocolate or vanilla powder	1 small banana	Option #2:		
	Option #4:	1 can of salmon or tuna on top of a garden salad		
1 small banana	apple			
1 teaspoon peanut butter	1 tablespoon peanut butter	1-2 tablespoons of olive oil and vinegar dressing		
(see *FIT 365* recipes)	Option #5:			
Option #3:	Any of the power snack recipes			
1 cup Greek yogurt				
1 cup berries				
Option #4:				
breakfast bowl				
(see *Layered Breakfast Bowl* recipe)				
Option #5:				
1 cup of steel-cut				

oatmeal (cooked) 1 scoop chocolate or vanilla FIT 365 1 small banana ¼ cup raisins (Mix together in a bowl)				

Appendix 7: Serving Size Guide

Visual Serving Size Guide

SERVING SIZE	VISUAL SERVING SIZE
CARBS	
1 cup raw veggies or medium piece or cup fruit	Tennis Ball
½ cup cooked veggies, fruit or juice	Golf Ball
1 oz. dried fruit	Golf Ball
$1/_3$ cup rice	Golf Ball
½ cup oatmeal, Cream of Wheat or noodles	Tennis Ball
PROTEINS	
3 oz. cooked chicken, beef or fish	iPod
1 oz. sliced deli meat	DVD
1 egg or 3 egg whites	Golf Ball
1 cup milk (cow, almond, coconut or hemp)	Baseball
1 cup yogurt	Tennis Ball
¼ cup cottage cheese	Baseball
HEALTHY FATS AND OILS	
¼ cup nuts	Ping Pong Ball
2 tablespoons nut butter	Ping Pong Ball

1 teaspoon oil	Marble
1 tablespoon dressing, sauce, butter or 5 olives	Quarter
1 ½ oz. cheese	3 Marbles
¼ avocado	Golf Ball
DESSERTS AND SWEETS	
1 slice cake or pie	iPod
1 scoop ice cream	Tennis Ball

DAILY SERVING RECOMMENDATIONS AND TIPS

CARBOHYDRATES

Vegetables

Key Points:

1. Eat at least 4-8 servings per day within 2-3 meals. Veggies should make up half of your plate.
2. 30% to 50% of your diet can easily come from carbohydrates in the form of vegetables and fruits.
3. Choose fresh or frozen vegetables instead of canned vegetables.
4. Eat roughly half of your vegetables raw when possible.
5. Steam vegetables to preserve nutrients and flavor.
6. Include dark green vegetables at least several times per week.
7. Starchy vegetables (corn, peas and potatoes) are counted as starch servings.

Fruits

Key Points:

1. Eat 1-4 servings a day. Eat less if you have been diagnosed with cancer, diabetes or hypoglycemia.
2. Choose fresh fruit rather than juice when possible for increased fiber.
3. When choosing juice, drink only pure juice with no added sugar or refined sweeteners.

Starches

Key Points:

1. Eat 0-2 servings a day. Eat less if you have body fat loss goals and for optimal health.
2. Starchy vegetables should make up your primary starch servings.
3. Keep starch exchanges from cereals (besides oatmeal), breads, pasta and starchy snack foods as limited as possible. Save them mostly for your Hour to Devour™ meals. All starchy foods are "glycemic" foods, meaning that they turn to sugar rapidly in the body.
4. Avoid processed starches, gluten and all "white starches" when possible.

   Note: Gluten intolerance affects 1 in every 133 Americans.

Gluten-free starches: potato, rice, corn, peas, oats, buckwheat, millet, nut flours, tapioca, amaranth, bean and sorghum

Starches with gluten: wheat, rye, couscous, kamut, spelt, barley, quinoa, triticale and semolina

Proteins

Key Points:

1. Eat 2-4 servings per meal depending on your size, amount of lean muscle mass, amount of physical activity and fitness goals.
2. Whey, egg, dairy and meats (in that order) have the highest Bio-Availability. These protein sources are the most usable by the body. Vegetable proteins (nuts, veggies and beans) have the lowest.
3. Avoid all non-fermented soy products (nearly all soy protein products except miso, tempeh, natto and tamari)
4. You don't need to avoid red meat as long as it's lean. Red meat is a good source of iron and zinc—minerals which many people need more of.
5. If you choose to avoid animal meat, you can use whey or egg white protein powder, cheese and eggs to meet your protein needs.
6. Use cooking methods that don't add fat—baking, broiling or grilling. Use wine or broth for poaching and stir-frying.

Dairy Products and Dairy Substitutes

Key Points:

1. Eat 0-3 servings per day.
2. Consider cheese a fat serving and use it sparingly as a sauce.
3. Consider yogurt and cottage cheese a protein serving.
4. Coconut milk, almond milk and hemp milk are the best milk substitutes.
5. Use non-pasteurized dairy products whenever possible.

Healthy Fats and Oils

Key Points:

1. Eat roughly 2-5 servings per day depending on your size, amount of lean muscle mass, amount of physical activity, fitness goals and the fat content of your protein sources. For example, eating higher fat protein sources like beef or salmon will require fewer fat sources throughout the day.

2. All fats are high in calories and should be consumed in moderation.
3. Avoid hydrogenated fats, partially hydrogenated oils and trans-fatty acids whenever possible.
4. Ensure your diet consists of enough omega-3 fatty acids. Supplement with cod liver, fish, krill or flaxseed oil.

Beverages

Key Points:

1. Drink 1 ounce of water per every pound of body weight (i.e. 100 lb. kid = 100 ounces)
2. Drinking empty calories is the easiest way to ruin your nutrition program as well as your fat loss goals. Most drinks besides water, coconut water and protein shakes should be kept to your Hour to Devour™.
3. Cut out caffeinated beverages as much as possible. You may include one caffeinated beverage per day. Once you start eating right, exercising and drinking enough water, you won't need caffeine. Try to switch to green tea instead of soda or coffee.
4. You can add lemon, lime, celery, cucumber or fruit to your water for flavor, along with a natural sweetener like Xylitol or Stevia. You can also add vitamin B or C powder.
5. Try to eliminate all soda, especially diet soda, from your diet completely, as it contains artificial sweeteners, phosphoric acid and carbonation that deplete calcium from your bones, and contains many other harmful substances.

Appendix 8: Healthy, Quick and Easy Recipes

Super morning starters, power snacks, healthy sauces and dressings, satisfying salads, amazing protein dishes, and super side dishes from Minh's Healthy Kitchen

SUPER MORNING STARTERS

Quick Scramblers

3 whole eggs

½ onion, diced

½ red pepper, diced

1 cup spinach, chopped

1 T coconut oil

Sea salt and pepper to taste

Melt oil in skillet and add onions to sauté.

In separate bowl, mix eggs, peppers, and spinach.

Pour contents of bowl into the skillet and scramble for 2-3 minutes.

Serve with pepper and salt if needed.

Layered Breakfast Bowl

Coconut, goat, or Greek yogurt

Cottage cheese

Berries

Pineapple or papaya

Raw honey

In a bowl, add ½ cup cottage cheese.

Add pineapple or papaya chunks.

Add ½ cup yogurt of choice.

Top with berries and 1 T of raw honey.

FIT 365® Recipes

FIT 365® Chocolate or Vanilla Peanut/Almond Butter

2 scoops chocolate or vanilla FIT 365®

1 T peanut or almond butter

1 small banana (optional)

6 to 8 oz. cold water, milk, almond milk, or coconut milk

5 ice cubes

Blend to smooth consistency and enjoy!

FIT 365® Banana Berry

2 scoops chocolate or vanilla FIT 365®

1 small banana

1/2 cup strawberries, blueberries or raspberries

6 to 8 oz. cold water, milk, almond milk, or coconut milk

5 ice cubes

Blend to smooth consistency and enjoy!

POWER SNACKS

Cottage cheese and pineapple or papaya

Hardboiled eggs and hummus

Banana and natural peanut butter

Sliced apples and raw almond butter

Yogurt with raspberries or blueberries and raw honey

Hummus and raw veggies

Celery, carrots, cauliflower, or broccoli with peanut butter or other raw nut butter

Cottage cheese with pineapple, papaya and cucumbers

Hardboiled eggs with hummus and mustard

Veggies and peanut butter

Raw nuts and dried fruits (almonds, walnuts, brazil nuts and figs, dates, apricots or raisins)

Protein Oatmeal Balls

1 cup organic oatmeal

1/3 cup raw honey

3 scoops FIT 365®

1 cup dry coconut

1/3 cup cocoa powder

½ cup boiling water

½ cup raisins

1 tsp vanilla extract

Place all dry ingredients in mixing bowl and mix.

Add boiling water.

Mix all ingredients together with spatula or use a mixer.

Form 1-inch balls and coat with cocoa.

Raw Nuts and Dried Fruit

Mix 1 cup of raw almonds, walnuts, pecans, brazil nuts, or pistachios and ½ cup of dried figs, raisins, or apricots in a food processor.

Form 1 inch cubes.

Note: You can also make your own variety mix. Just throw your favorite nuts and dried fruit in a bag.

HEALTHY SAUCES AND DRESSINGS

These sauces and dressings are simple to make and go with almost anything you put on your plate. They make everything flavorful and healthy!

Use my five "S" acronyms to remember how to balance my dressings:

Sweet – raw honey, stevia

Salty – liquid aminos (nama shoyu), sea salt

Sour – juice of lime, lemon, apple cider vinegar, balsamic vinegar

Spicy – garlic, ginger, onions

Savory – extra virgin olive oil, avocado, tahini

Sweet Balsamic Basil Dressing

1/3 cup extra virgin olive oil

Pinch of stevia

½ cup balsamic vinegar

½ cup fresh basil

¼ cup raspberries or pomegranate

1 T ginger

3 cloves garlic

1/3 cup lemon juice

Mix in blender and enjoy!

Italian Dressing

1/3 cup extra virgin olive oil

1 T dried parsley

½ cup fresh basil

4 cloves garlic

4 T apple cider vinegar or balsamic vinegar

½ cup lemon juice

1 T organic Italian seasoning

Pinch of stevia

½ tsp sea salt

Mix in blender and enjoy!

Goat Cheese Pesto Sauce

4 cup fresh basil

1 cup fresh parsley

1/3 cup extra virgin olive oil

½ cup pine nuts

2 oz of raw goat feta

½ cup sundried tomatoes

Mix in food processor on "pulse" setting.

Curry Sauce

1 ½ cup coconut milk

½ cup chicken broth

1 T red curry paste

1/3 cup natural organic peanut butter, crunchy

2 T lime juice

2 tsp honey

Mix all ingredients in a bowl and pour it over any sautéed chicken or meat dishes.

Mango Sauce

1 mango, peeled and seeded

1 T dried thyme

3 T balsamic vinegar

2-3 cloves garlic

1 tsp sea salt

Pepper to taste

Mix in blender and enjoy!

Lemon Mint Tzatziki

1 cup goat yogurt

1 medium cucumber, diced

2 tsp lemon juice

1 tsp garlic, minced

½ tsp lemon zest

1 T mint leaves, minced

1 tsp extra virgin olive oil

Mix in blender and enjoy!

Lemon Yogurt Spread

1 cup Greek yogurt

1 T Dijon mustard

Juice of 1 lemon

1 tsp paprika

Sea salt and ground pepper to taste

In a small bowl, mix all ingredients and enjoy with fish, chicken or veggies.

SATISFYING SALADS

No more boring iceberg lettuce and tomato salads! Salads can be both fun and simple to make! Explore your creative side and experiment with all different kinds of healthy veggies and fruits. There are literally hundreds of veggie, fruit, meat, and sauce combinations you can try. Here are some go-to salads that will leave you satisfied.

My Big Greek Salad

Arugula

Cherry tomatoes

Red peppers

White kidney beans

Artichoke hearts

Olives

Red onions

Fennel

Parsley

Basil

Avocado chunks

Recommended: Italian dressing

Spinach, Apple, and Goat Cheese Salad

Spinach

Apple

Goat cheese

Walnuts

Red onions

Recommended: Sweet balsamic basil dressing

AMAZING PROTEIN DISHES

Roasted Halibut (serves 4)

2 lbs halibut

2/3 cup mango or spicy tomato salsa

1/3 cup Dijon mustard

2 T chopped parsley

1 T lemon juice

Preheat oven to 425.

Combine salsa, mustard, parsley and lemon in small bowl.

Cut 4 pieces of foil into 12" squares.

Arrange fish in center of foil and spoon 1-1 ½ T sauce over fish. Fold and place on cookie sheet.

Bake 8-10 minutes, serve remaining sauce separately.

Wild Salmon w/ Bok Choy (serves 4)

4-5 oz salmon filets

4 heads baby bok choy, cleaned and leaves separated

1 cup baby bella mushrooms

3 scallions, thinly sliced

2 tsp fresh ginger, minced

8 T fresh squeezed orange juice

3 tsp honey

1 tsp Dijon mustard

1 tsp orange peel

¼ tsp ground coriander

Preheat oven to 425.

In a bowl, mix orange juice, ginger, honey, mustard, orange peel, and coriander.

Place bok choy in a baking dish and put the salmon on top.

Drizzle the mix over the salmon.

Cover with foil and bake for 15 minutes.

Meat and Veggie Stew

1 lb healthy lean ground meat (could be grass fed beef/turkey/chicken)

2 T coconut oil

1 onion, diced

1 yellow pepper, diced

1 red pepper, diced

1 ½ cup organic tomato puree

2 cup chicken broth

4 cloves minced garlic

12 pitted olives

1/3 cup capers

4 medium diced sweet potatoes

1 lb sweet peas

1 tsp sea salt

1 T cumin

1 T chili powder

2 T dried parsley

½ cup fresh cilantro

Put coconut oil in pan (preferably cast iron) to melt.

Add garlic and onions to sauté for 3-4 minutes.

Add ground meat and stir for another 5 minutes.

Add broth, dry spices, peppers, and sweet potatoes and cover for 10 minutes.

Add in the rest of the ingredients and cook over low to medium heat until done. Serve topped with fresh cilantro.

Turkey Burgers (serves 4)

1 lb ground organic turkey

1 clove garlic, minced

1 scallion, including green parts, sliced thin

2 T red bell pepper, chopped small

1 tsp fresh ginger, minced

½ cup fresh spinach, finely chopped

2 T apple cider vinegar

Sea salt and pepper

In a medium bowl, mix all ingredients.

Form into 4 patties and grill over medium heat until done, approximately 8 minutes per side.

Serve over any big leafy greens like Bibb lettuce, romaine, or Swiss chard. Top with sliced tomatoes, avocados, onions and one of the fantastic sauces in this book.

SUPER SIDE DISHES

Crisp Green Beans

1 lb French green beans

2 T coconut oil

3 tsp McCormick's Steakhouse seasoning, grinder

Preheat oven to 400 degrees.

Put coconut oil and seasoning in a pan (preferably cast iron) over burner until melted. Toss green beans in the oil and place in oven for 12-15 minutes or until crisp and tender.

Sautéed Kale

1 head organic kale, chopped small

1 medium onion, chopped

2 T coconut oil

2 T balsamic vinegar

1 ½ tsp sea salt

1 tsp fresh ground pepper

Add oil to skillet on medium high.

Add onions and sauté for 3 minutes.

Add kale and sauté for another 8 minutes.

Remove pan from the heat and add balsamic vinegar, salt and pepper to coat.

Blanched Asparagus

1 lb fresh asparagus spears, trimmed

2 tsp sea salt

Juice of 1 lemon

Fill a pot about ¾ full with water. Add salt and bring to boil.

Add in asparagus for no more than 3 minutes.

Remove and drain in a colander. Add ice to stop the cooking process.

Add fresh-squeezed lemon juice.

Recommended: Eat with lemon yogurt spread

Appendix 9: Restaurant Eating Simplified

GAME PLAN:

1. Choose a protein, carbohydrate, and occasionally add a fat source from the "Feel-good Choices" at each meal. Many protein sources already have enough fat.

2. Dietary carbohydrates are divided between the "Carbs" (fruits and vegetables) category and "Starch" category. Occasionally, feel free to add a "Starch" option to your meal. Note: Many times, if you eat enough in the "Carbs" category, you won't need to add any "Starch."

3. Save the "Not-So-Good Choices" for your Hour to Devour™ meals.

Breakfast

Feel-Good Choices	Not-So-Good Choices
• Protein—chicken, cottage cheese, eggs, omelets, steak and turkey • Carbs—fruit, spinach and tomatoes • Starch—corn tortillas, oatmeal and other whole-grain cereals, skillet potatoes, whole-grain bagels and whole grain breads • Fat—avocado and cheese	• Sugar cereals or processed/packaged baked goods like pastries, bagels, and breads

Steak and Seafood

Feel-Good Choices	Not-So-Good Choices
• Protein—all baked and grilled seafood, chicken and steak • Carbs—salads and vegetables • Starch—red potatoes, sweet potatoes and yams	• Bread, fried foods

Italian

Feel-Good Choices	Not-So-Good Choices
• Protein—fish, grilled chicken and lean beef • Carbs—salads and veggies • Fat—extra virgin olive oil and cheeses	• Bread, pasta and pizza

Mexican

Feel-Good Choices	Not-So-Good Choices
• Protein—grilled chicken, beef, fish and fajitas • Carbs—salad, grilled or cooked veggies and salsa • Starch—brown rice, black beans and wheat tortillas • Fat—guacamole	• Chips, fried food, refried beans, flour tortillas

Chinese, Japanese, Sushi, Thai, and Vietnamese

Feel-Good Choices	Not-So-Good Choices
• Protein—chicken, fish, turkey and beef • Carbs—vegetables and seaweed • Starch—baked egg rolls or spring rolls, brown rice and rice noodles. • Fats—light sauces	• Fried foods, non-fermented soy like tofu, noodle dishes and white rice

Greek

Feel-Good Choices	Not-So-Good Choices
• Protein—chicken, fish, turkey, lamb and beef • Carbs—Greek salad and vegetables • Fats—dressing, olives and cheese	• Bread and pitas

Indian

Feel-Good Choices	Not-So-Good Choices
• Protein—chicken, fish, turkey, lamb and beef • Carbs—vegetables • Starch—brown rice • Fats—coconut cream sauces	• Fried foods, dairy cream sauces, white rice, bread

Appendix 10: Fast Food Survival Guide

Let me start out by saying that I am NOT a fan of most fast food. Nearly all fast food is not "real" food. Fast food should be a last resort and is usually more expensive and takes more time than making a meal at home. For example, a typical value meal at a popular fast food chain including a burger, French fries, and a soft drink costs approximately $6.50. If you break down the cost per serving from a grocery store, you can buy and barbeque a chicken breast, a sweet potato, and a cup of steamed veggies for roughly $2. Moreover, fast food is not even fast! By the time you drive to a fast food restaurant, wait in line at the drive thru, and come home you could have made and enjoyed a home-cooked meal and even cleaned up the mess. If you become a conscious eater by planning your daily meals and learning how to cook quick and delicious recipes, you won't need to rely on fast food.

Let's be real: for most of us, there are times you're stuck in a bind and you need to go the fast food route. Here's a survival guide to the world of fast food so you'll feel confident knowing what you should choose and what you should avoid.

You know from reading this book that I'm not a fan of counting calories. Yet I want to show you through calorie content how you can make the best choices if you find yourself in a bind and need to go with fast food.

SIMPLIFY YOUR FOOD

Let's take a look at a popular fast-food chain here in Southern California called In N' Out Burger®. The classic order at this fast-food chain is the Double Double® combo meal. This "value" meal comes with a double patty hamburger, a soft drink, and a side of French fries. Check out how modifying your options and simplifying your food can significantly cut the amount of damage done from that fast food meal.

Double Double® combo meal with a Coke®: 1,268 calories, 44 grams of protein, 147 grams carbohydrates and 59 grams fat

Choose water instead of Coke®: SAVE 198 calories

Get rid of the fries: SAVE 400 calories

Replace the sauce with ketchup and mustard: SAVE 60 calories

Order "Protein Style" by replacing the bun with a lettuce wrap: SAVE 150 calories

NEW total caloric breakdown: 460 calories, 33 grams of protein, 13 grams of carbohydrates and 30 grams of fat

That's a savings of 808 calories! Calorically speaking, this means you could eat almost three "Protein Style" Double Doubles® with ketchup and mustard for every one Double Double® combo meal!

Tips for making the best choices at fast food restaurants:

Go lean! Choose leaner meats like chicken and turkey over beef. Most fast food burgers are low-quality, fatty beef that are pumped full of hormones.

Choose cleaner cooking styles. Frying will not only add unhealthy fat, sodium, and calories, but it will destroy the nutritional value of the food. Avoid words like deep-fried, creamy, crispy, or scalloped. Instead, choose words like baked, seared, steamed, boiled, barbequed or poached.

Deny the sides. Typical side dishes at fast food restaurants are fried and lack real nutrition. Choose a side salad or a piece of fruit whenever possible or simply avoid the sides. If you're still hungry when you get home, reach for a piece of fruit or some homemade trail mix.

Watch the sauce and dressings! House special sauces, sour cream, mayonnaise, and prepared salad dressings like blue cheese, ranch, or even some vinaigrettes can easily double your total caloric intake and are typically packed full of fat, sugar and salt. Instead, add healthy fats like avocado, a little cheese, or healthy dressings like olive oil and vinegar. On sandwiches, stick with mustard.

Don't drink your calories! Soda is a huge source of hidden calories. Choose water with lemon or unsweetened tea and break your addiction to soft drinks. Make sure you drink a bunch of water before your meal, as it will keep your appetite in check. Remember, when you think you're hungry, you may be thirsty, and when you think you're thirsty you're already dehydrated.

Eat like a turtle, not a racehorse. Slow down and savor your food. Chew each bite thoroughly and allow time for your body to tell you when it's content. It takes 20 minutes for your body to tell your mind it's full [1]. You'll eat less and digest your food better. You'll walk away full and satisfied, not stuffed and bloated.

Appendix 11: You are What You Eat

Society has lost sight of looking at food as nutrition, and replaced it with the mistake of viewing food as calories. Most Americans eat plenty of calories, but not enough nutrients. This is due to poor nutrition education, lack of self-discipline, and addiction to high-sugar and high-starch processed foods.

Throughout history, leading scholars have understood that real food is nature's medicine. Fruits, vegetables, and herbs contain nutrients that can keep you healthy. In 431 B.C., the father of Western medicine, Hippocrates, proclaimed, "Let thy food be thy medicine and thy medicine be thy food." In 300 C.E., The Talmud unveiled the wisdom that certain fruits and vegetables look like parts of the human body that they benefit. While these foods have multiple nutritional benefits, here's a little look into the beauty of food and its medicinal power.

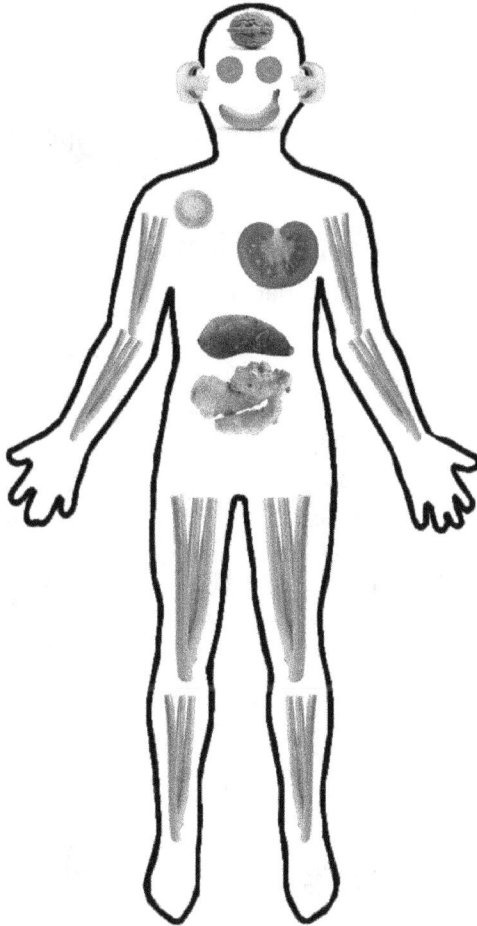

IF IT LOOKS LIKE YOU IT'S GOOD FOR YOU!

FOOD:	LOOKS LIKE:	CONTAINS/GOOD FOR:
Carrot (sliced)	Eyes (pupil, iris, and radiating lines)	Vitamin A = Blood flow to and function of the eyes [39]
Walnut	Brain	Omega-3 fatty acids =

		Develop neurotransmitters to support healthy brain function [40]
Tomato	Heart (red w/four chambers)	Lycopene = Healthy heart, reduces risk of heart disease [41]
Grapes	Hang in cluster shape of heart, look like blood cells	Resveratrol = Cardiovascular food that prevents heart disease [42]
Celery	Bones	Silicon and Vitamin K = Good for bone strength; all made up of 23% sodium, same as bones [43]
Sweet Potatoes/Yams	Pancreas	Balance glycemic index for diabetics [44]
Banana	Smile	Tryptophan = Raises mood enhancing hormone serotonin [45]
Ginger	Stomach	Helps with digestion, stomachaches, and nausea [46]
Mushroom	Ear	Vitamin D = Bone health, even tiny ones in ear that transmit

		sound to brain [47]
Onions (sliced)	Cells	Quercetin = Helps clear waste materials from all of the body's cells (48)

EAT FOOD THAT LOOKS HOW YOU WANT TO LOOK

Here is your quick tip guide to knowing if a type of food is good for you:

I WANT TO LOOK:	**I WILL EAT:**
Lean, fit, toned	Lean animal protein
Healthy	Variety of vegetables, especially green veggies
Bright and full of energy	Fruits and berries
Strong	Nuts, seeds and healthy oils

I DON'T WANT TO LOOK:	**I WILL LIMIT:**
Fat	Fatty animal protein
Greasy or oily	Fried foods
Soft and squishy	White bread, doughnuts, cake or pastries
Phony, fake or tired	Candy, sweets, ice cream

Appendix 12: Hour to Devour

The Hour to Devour™ is a planned meal once or maybe twice a week where you "go to town" and eat ANYTHING you've been craving that doesn't move (and isn't poisonous/toxic... although in actuality, they are :). This can include ice cream, pizza, pasta, candy, fast food or other bread products. This is the hour when you look at the menu and say, "Yes, please!"*

*Warning: Overindulgence usually leads to initial joy followed by regret in the form of upset stomach, lethargy, gas, bloating, and a multitude of other temporary symptoms that just "aren't fun." The Hour to Devour™ is not included in the program of diabetics, gastric bypass clients, heart patients, anyone with severe food allergies, celiac disease, or anyone with an exceptionally weak immune system. Make sure you consult a physician before incorporating an Hour to Devour™ into your eating plan.

Why incorporate The Hour to Devour™ into your healthy lifestyle?

- It eliminates the diet mentality
- It keeps you "human"
- It helps set weekly objectives
- It prevents you from "falling off the health wagon"
- It improves awareness of how different foods affect your body

The Hour to Devour™ can remain part of someone's program even after they have reached their weight loss goals. Most people start out overindulging during their hour but quickly learn that all they need is a small indulgence—like a piece of pizza or a small ice cream cone—to keep them from feeling deprived of their favorite foods and committed to a healthy lifestyle.

Appendix 13: The Playground Workout

"I never set out to be a Hall of Fame baseball player or Hall of Fame football player. I just loved to play. Period." –Bo Jackson, Hall of Fame athlete, MLB and NFL

NOTE: FREE EXERCISE VIDEO DEMONSTRATIONS ARE AVAILABLE AT WWW.THEZEBRABOOK.COM

No excuses! Your body is the only equipment you need. You can do this workout at home, in a field, at a playground... anywhere! You are your own gym! And best of all, it's going to be *fun*!

You don't need weights to sculpt the physique of a champion. Whether you want to build muscle or develop a lean body, you already have the tools you need. Take Bo Jackson, for example. Bo is known as one of the greatest athletes of all time. He was the first athlete to be named an all-star in two major sports (baseball and football) and also won the Heisman trophy in 1985.

Yet what many people don't know about Bo is that this 6-foot 1-inch, 225-pound physical specimen built his physique using only his body as a gym. Bo grew up dirt poor as the eighth of ten children and didn't have the luxury of joining a gym or having his own set of weights. According to Bo, he and his siblings "never had enough food." His mother struggled to make ends meet as a housekeeper and a single mother.

Despite all these challenges, Bo had an incredible work ethic. His mother was a fantastic role model, as she believed that Bo needed to give education at least as much effort as sports. She made sure he always put his education first. He needed to have A's in order to play school sports. In addition to his tremendous natural ability, it was sports and excellent grades that allowed him to get into college at Auburn and led him out of poverty.

Even though he was drafted into Major League Baseball before he graduated and had a Hall of Fame career in both baseball and football, Bo continues to live the life of a true champion. He understands the value of higher education. Upon retiring from sports, he kept the promise he made to his mother before she died of cancer in 1992 and went back to Auburn, and graduated with a Bachelor of Science degree in Family and Childhood Development. [49]

Not only is Bo a great athlete, he is also a great human being. He lives the championship lifestyle by giving back to the community as CEO of the Bo Jackson Elite Sports Complex near Chicago and President of the Sports Medicine Council, a non-profit youth outreach organization owned by HealthSouth.

Bo is also a testament to the fact that mindset is everything when it comes to sports and exercise. Just like anything else in life, you have to combine a positive attitude and hard work to achieve your goals. According to Bo, "It's all about the attitude, gut, heart and determination to go out and give 120% every time." [50]

Exercise doesn't have to be about monitoring numbers like weight, reps and sets or heart rate, time and incline. Instead, find a physical activity or a sport you're passionate about, then get out there and play every day! Just like Bo lived in the moment and focused on enjoying playing, you too can develop a mindset of getting off the couch and having fun being fit rather than forcing yourself to do boring, monotonous workouts.

Challenge yourself to try something new and you'll be surprised what you can achieve with a little practice, and how much fun it can be!

GO TO WWW.THEZEBRABOOK.COM AND WATCH SOME OF OUR FREE EXERCISE AND GAME DEMONSTRATIONS.

Follow along with the qualified fitness professionals and simply challenge yourself to complete these exercises with good form.

Body Weight Exercises

Instructions:

Pick two exercises from each category to create two rounds.

Try this workout as an example:

Round 1: Push-ups with rotations ⇨ ice skaters ⇨ bicycle crunches ⇨ mountain climbers ⇨ child pose

Round 2: Bear crawls ⇨ squats jumps ⇨ plank ⇨ sprint in place ⇨ downward dog

Upper Body		
Push-ups	Push-ups with Rotations	Plyo Push-ups
Walking Push-ups	Tricep Push-ups	Bear Crawls
Tabletops	Pull-ups	

Lower Body		
Lunges	Side Lunges	Power Lunges
Plyo Lunges	Lunges with Rotation	Squats
Squat Jumps	Ice Skaters	

Core		
Planks	Side Planks	Moving Planks
Reverse Crunches	Bicycle Crunches	Oblique Crunches

Cardio Mix Up		
Mountain Climbers	Sprinting in Place	Jogging
Sprints	Interval Training	Skipping

Swimming	Spinning	Biking
Jumping Rope	Trampoline	Boxing

Yoga Stretches		
Child Pose	Downward Dog	Tree Pose
Sun Salutations	Cat/Cow	Warrior 2

CITATIONS:

1. www.collegesportsscholarships.com/percentage-high-school-athletes-ncaa-college.htm
2. sportsillustrated.cnn.com/vault/article/magazine/MAG11 53364/1/index.htm
3. www.nfl.com, www.nba.com, www.nhl.com, www.mlb.com
4. Cordain, Loren. *The Paleo Diet: Lose Weight and Get Healthy by Eating the Food You Were Designed to Eat.* New York: Wiley. 2002
5. Colby, J.J., et al. "Promoting the selection of healthy food through menu item description in a family-style restaurant." *American Journal of Preventative Medicine*, 1987. 3(3): p. 171-7.
6. Lorson B. Melgar-Quinonez, and H. Taylor, C. "Correlates of fruit and vegetable intake in US children." *Journal of the American Dietetic Association,* 2009;109:474-478.
7. Mercola, Dr. Joseph and Degen Pearsall, Dr. Kendra. *Sweet Deception: Why Splenda, NutraSweet, and the FDA May Be Hazardous to Your Health.* Thomas Nelson Inc. 2006.
8. Lockwood, Sophie. "Zebras." *Children's World, Inc.* 2008
9. "Zebra." The Gale Encyclopedia of Science. 2008
10. Schaller, George. "The Serengeti Lion: A Study of Predator-Prey Relations." *Wildlife Behavior and Ecology series.* University of Chicago Press. 1976.
11. www.bloomberg.com/apps/news?pid=newsarchive&sid= aAyTBdCuTgWM&refer=healthcare
12. Ma, Unsheng and Bertone, Elizabeth. "Association between Eating Patterns and Obesity in a Free-living US Adult

Population." *American Journal of Epidemiology.* July 2003;158: 85-92.

13. Vanderwal, J.S., Gupta, A., Khosla, P., and Dhurandhar, N.V. "Egg Breakfast Enhances Weight Loss." *International Journal of Obesity (London).* 2008 August 5; 32 (10) 1545-51.

14. Fulgoni III, Victor L. "Current Protein Intake in America: Analysis of the National Health and Nutrition Examination Survey, 2003-2004."*American Journal of Clinical Nutrition.* May 2008; 87(5): 1554S=1557S

15. FAO. "Amino Acid Content of Foods." FAO Nutritional Studies No. 24, 1970.

16. Droge, W., and Breitkreutz R. "Glutathione and immune function." Proceedings of the Nutritional Society November 2000 Nov; 59 (4): 595-600.

17. Carpenter, Dr. Dave. *Change Your Water, Change Your Life.* Enagic USA, Inc.

18. Institute of Medicine. "Dietary reference intakes for water, potassium, sodium, chloride and sulfate." The National Academic Press: Washington, 2004

19. "Caffeine Content of Beverages, Foods, & Medications." The Vaults of Erowid. July 7, 2006. Retrieved 2009-08-03.

20. Mayo Clinic staff. "Caffeine content for coffee, tea, soda and more". Mayo Clinic. Retrieved 2010-11-08.

21. Mattes, R.D. "Physiologic responses to sensory stimulation by food: nutritional implications." *Journal of the American Dietetic Association*. 1997; 97:406–13.

22. Fowler, S.P. 65th Annual Scientific Sessions, American Diabetes Association, San Diego, June 10-14, 2005; Abstract 1058-P. Sharon P. Fowler, MPH, University of Texas Health Science Center School of Medicine, San Antonio. Leslie Bonci, MPH, RD, director, sports nutrition, University of Pittsburgh Medical Center.

23. Fefe, Bruce, ND. *Coconut Water For Health and Healing*. Piccadilly Books, Ltd.: Colorado, 2008.

24. Johnson, R.J. and Gower, T. "The Sugar Fix: The High-Fructose Fallout That is Making You Sick and Fat." Pocket, 416 pp. 2009.

25. Michaud, D. "Dietary Sugar, Glycemic Load, and Pancreatic Cancer Risk in a Prospective Study." *Journal of the National Cancer Institute*. Sep 4, 2002; 94 (17):1293-300.

26. Christensen, L., et al. "Impact of a Dietary Change on Emotional Distress." *Journal of Abnormal Psychology*.1985;94(4):565-79.

27. Relser, S. "Effects of Sugars on Indices on Glucose Tolerance to Humans." *American Journal of Clinical Nutrition*. 1986:43;151-159.

28. Goldman, J., et al. "Behavioral Effects of Sucrose on Preschool Children." *Journal of Abnormal Child Psychology*. 1986;14(4):565-577.

29. Molteni, R., et al. "A High-fat, Refined Sugar Diet Reduces Hippocampal Brain-derived Neurotrophic Factor, Neuronal Plasticity, and Learning." *Neuroscience.* 2002;112(4): 803-814.

30. O'Brien, R. and Kranz, R. *The Unhealthy Truth: How our food is making us sick and what we can do about it.* Broadway Books: New York, 2009.

31. Salatin, J. *Pastured Poultry Profits.* Polyface, Inc.: Virginia, 1996.

32. Massiera, F., Barbry, P., Guesnet, P., Joly, A., Luquet, S., Brest, C.M., Mohsen-Kanson, T., Amri, E., and Ailhaud, G. "A Western-like fat diet is sufficient to induce a gradual enhancement in fat mass over generations." *Journal of Lipid Research.* 51:2352-2361. 2010.

33. Hoff, J., Gran, A., and Helgerud, J. "Maximal strength training improves aerobic endurance performance." *Scandinavian Journal Medical Science in Sports.* 2002 Oct;12(5):288-95.

34. Tanaka, H., Costill, D.L., Thomas, R., Fink, W.J., and Widrick, J.J. (1993). "Dry-land resistance training for competitive swimming." *Medicine and Science in Sports and Exercise.* 25, 952-959.

35. Fleck, S.J., and Kraemer, W.J. *Designing Resistance Training Programs: 3rd Edition.* Human Kinetics: Champaign, IL, 2004.

36. Marklein, Mary Beth. "Today's Freshmen Want To Lend A Hand." *USA Today.* January 26, 2006.

37. Mindful Awareness Research Center at University of California Los Angeles (http://marc.ucla.edu).

38. Dweck, Carol S. *Mindset: The New Psychology of Success.* Random House, 2006.

39. Agricultural Marketing Resource Center (AgMRC). Carrot Profile. 2011; Iowa State University, Ames, IO. (http://www.agmrc.org)

40. Marangoni, F., Colombo, C., Martiello, A., Poli, A., Paoletti, R., and Galli, C. "Levels of the n-3 fatty acid eicosapentaenoic acid in addition to those of alpha linolenic acid are sign,ificantly raised in blood lipids by the intake of four walnuts a day in humans." *Nutrition for Metabolic Cardiovascular Disease.* 2006 September 25; [Epub ahead of print] 2006. PMID:17008073.

41. Wood, M. "Tangerine Tomatoes Top Reds in Preliminary Lycopene Study." *Agricultural Research.* Washington: Feb 2011. Vol. 59, Issue 2; p. 15. 2011.

42. Bertelli, A.A., and Das, D.K. "Grapes, wines, resveratrol, and heart health." *Journal of Cardiovascular Pharmacology.* 2009 Dec; 54(6):468-76. 2009.

43. McKeith, Gillian. *You Are What You Eat: The Plan That Will Change Your Life.* Barnes and Noble, 2004.

44. Bahado-Singh, P.S., Wheatley, A.O., et al. "Food processing methods influence the glycemic indices of some commonly eaten West Indian carbohydrate-rich foods." *British Journal of Nutrition.* 2006 Sep;96(3):476-81. 2006.

45. http://nutritiondata.self.com/facts/fruits-and-fruit-juices/1846/2

46. Borrelli, F., Capasso, R., Aviello, G., Pittler, M.H., and Izzo, A.A. "Effectiveness and safety of ginger in the treatment of pregnancy-induced nausea and vomiting." *Obstetric Gynecology*. 2005 April; 105(4):849-56. 2005. PMID:15802416.

47. Koyyalamudi, S.R., Jeong, S.C., and Song, C.H., et al. "Vitamin D2 formation and bioavailability from Agaricus bisporus button mushrooms treated with ultraviolet irradiation." *Journal of Agricultural Food Chemistry*. 2009 April 22;57(8):3351-5. 2009.

48. Smith, Crystal, Lombard, Kevin A., Peffley, Ellen B., and Liu, Weixin. "Genetic Analysis of Quercetin in Onion (Allium cepa L.) Lady Raider". *The Texas Journal of Agriculture and Natural Resource (Agriculture Consortium of Texas)*. 2003; 16: 24–8.

49. "Bo Jackson—Growing Up" (http://sports.jrank.org/pages/2225/Jackson-Bo-Growing-Up.html)

50. "Interview with Bo Jackson." National Strength and Conditioning Association. Retrieved October 5, 2009.

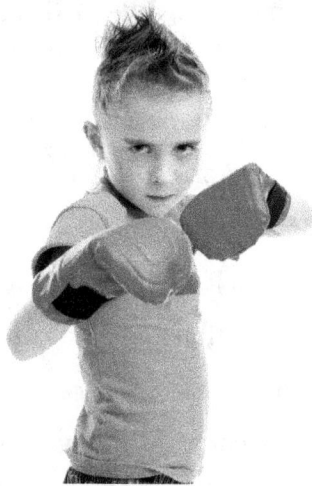

DRINK A SHAKE & FIGHT

CHILDHOOD OBESITY!

A percentage of all FIT 365® shake orders is donated to organizations including National PAL (Police Athletics/Activities League) and the Del Mar Carmel Valley Sharks to help fight childhood obesity.

PAL uses this money for our Strive 4 Fitness® program to help kids across the nation learn that living a healthy lifestyle is not about being perfect, but about doing your best every day, having pride in yourself, and striving to make your community a better place.

The Del Mar/Carmel Valley Sharks use this money to provide scholarships for kids who cannot afford to play soccer in their leagues and camps.

By simply drinking FIT 365® as part of your healthy lifestyle, you are helping us provide kids with the resources they need to be their best.

ABOUT PAL (POLICE ATHLETICS/ACTIVITIES LEAGUES)

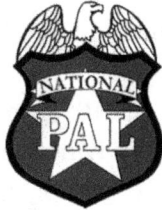

"The Strive 4 Fitness® *Live Like a Champion* kids program shows you that becoming a champion and living a healthy lifestyle is not an overnight fix but a process. It is not about being perfect, but about doing your best every day, having pride in yourself, and striving to make your community a better place to live." – Michael D. Dillhyon, Executive Director of National PAL

Police Athletic/Activities Leagues (PAL) is a safe and affordable kids program led by police officers and civilians that has proven to prevent crime and improve relations between police, kids and communities.

The PAL model was developed in 1914 in New York City, NY, in response to rising juvenile delinquency. The New York City Police Department recognized that their efforts to provide safe and positive activities for youth reduced the likelihood that they would participate in delinquent behavior. Recognizing the value of that first PAL program in the boroughs of New York City, other communities began to develop their own PAL Program. Serving approximately 1.5 million youth in communities across the country, today's PAL Chapters provide opportunities for youth to participate in a variety of activities, including athletics, recreation, education and community service programs.

To support the collective efforts of PAL Chapters across the country, The National Association of Police Athletic/Activities Leagues, Inc. (National PAL) was formed in 1940. Through the years, National PAL has provided local PAL Chapters with financial and programmatic resources. The value of the PAL model has been recognized by other organizations across the country. Today, National PAL is a member of the United States Olympic Committee Multi-Sports Organization and USA Boxing. Other organizations have partnered with National PAL throughout the years, including the Cal Ripken, Sr. Foundation, USA Football, US Soccer Foundation, NFL, NBA, NHL and many other national organizations.

Many champions have gotten their start at a PAL Chapter, including Muhammad Ali, Harvey Schiller, Congressman Frank Wolf, Boomer Esiason, Nick Lowry, Larry Holmes, Evander Holyfield and Bill Cosby.

ABOUT THE DEL MAR CARMEL VALLEY SHARKS

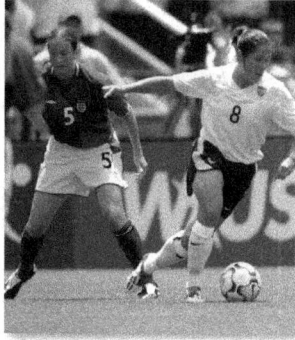

Photo by Michael Stahlschmidt

"Never give up! During my twelve-year career with the U.S. Women's National Team, I had many roles. I was a starter, I was dubbed the "super sub," and I was even cut from the team. It would have been easy to give up and walk away, but I chose to fight. In 1996 I was cut from the Olympic team but instead of giving up, I worked twice as hard and eventually not only earned a spot on the roster of 16 to represent the US at the Atlanta Olympics, but also was a starter and finished the tournament as the leading scorer. You have to always believe in yourself and learn to embrace the challenge. When things are hard, you learn to appreciate and enjoy the successes even more! The World Championship and the gold medals are cherished, but what I cherish more are the friends I made along the way and the life lessons I was able to ex-tract from the wins as well as the challenges. The Strive 4 Fitness® *Live Like a Champion* kids program is all about challenging yourself to achieve your true potential."

— Shannon MacMillan, Director of Competitive Programs for the DMCV Sharks, U.S. Olympic Gold Medalist, Women's Soccer, 1999

Women's World Cup Champion, twelve-year career with US Women's National Team with 176 games, 1995 Hermann Trophy Winner, Best Female Collegiate Soccer Player

The DMCV Sharks is a nonprofit, volunteer organization that has been serving the San Diego suburban community of Carmel Valley since its inception in 1980. The Sharks league offers recreational programs, competitive programs and camps for players of all abilities. The Sharks organization is one of the largest soccer leagues in the country and delivers a quality soccer experience each year to thousands of kids, ages five to nineteen.

The club regularly contends for championships in state and regional soccer tournaments in all age groups. The hallmark of all DMCV Sharks' teams is superb individual skills. Development of the individual player is emphasized over team success. However, winning is a natural consequence of maximizing each individual player's potential. Players are given equal playing time in league games and are encouraged to pursue their highest individual goals.

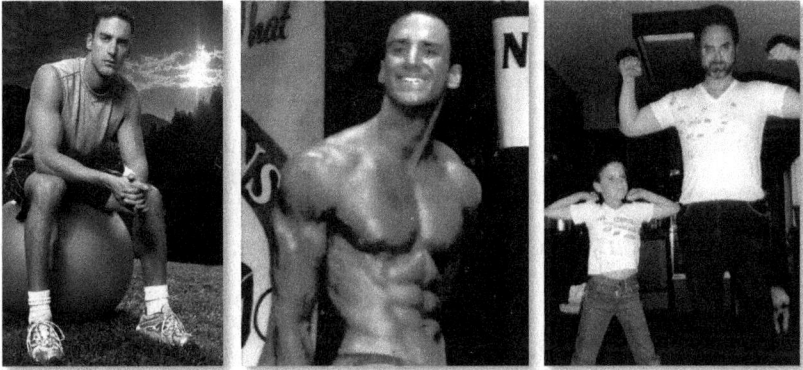

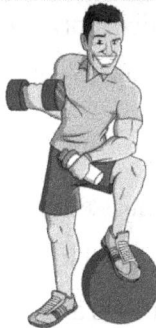

"Me, Coach Kyle"

KYLE BROWN

BA, CCN, CSCS, YFS, CMTA, NASM-CPT

Celebrity Personal Trainer, Nutritionist, Author, Speaker, and Inventor

Kyle Brown is a health and nutrition expert whose portfolio includes everything from leading workshops for Fortune 500 companies and authoring articles in top-ranked fitness journals to training celebrity clientele, from pro and Olympic athletes to CEOs to multi-platinum recording artists. In 2010 and 2011, he was voted San Diego's Best Personal Trainer by the readers of *The San Diego Union Tribune* and www.SignOnSanDiego.com. In 2012, Kyle can be seen as the co-host nutrition expert on Fox Sports Network's "I Wanna Be A World Class Athlete!" television show.

Kyle's holistic approach to health and fitness ensures that your body is given everything it requires to maintain health and build vitality from the inside out. Kyle specializes in customizing healthy nutrition and personal training programs based around your body's unique biochemistry as well as your on-the-go lifestyle. His versatile personal training programs incorporate everything from whole-body integration to bodybuilding-style resistance training and Muay Thai (Thai kickboxing).

Kyle is the CEO of Strive 4 Fitness® and creator of FIT 365®, an all-natural, complete low-calorie meal in a shake (www.Fit365.com). FIT 365® is completely nutritious and incredibly delicious. Each shake you drink helps fight childhood obesity, as a portion of proceeds goes to support organizations combating childhood obesity.

After a decade of training the elite, Kyle has committed himself to joining the fight against childhood obesity. In his new book, entitled *How Much Does A Zebra Weigh?* , Kyle, a certified youth fitness specialist, has developed a revolutionary game plan to make living a healthy lifestyle fun and exciting for young people. Kyle has partnered with organizations including National PAL (Police Athletics/Activities League) and travels across the nation to speak to kids and teens and implement his program.

Degrees and Certifications:

BA in Journalism, Indiana University

CCN: Certified Clinical Nutritionist

CSCS: Certified Strength and Conditioning Specialist

YFS: Youth Fitness Specialist

CMTA: Certified Metabolic Typing Advisor

NASM-CPT: Certified Personal Trainer

PTA Global: Completed Bridging Course

ViPR: Certified ViPR Instructor

CBTI: Cross-Box Training Instructor

EFI Sports Medicine: Gravity Certified Instructor

TRX Certified Suspension Training Instructor

Notable:

Co-host nutrition expert on Fox Sports Network's "I Wanna Be A World Class Athlete!" television show.

Educational video on Youtube.com has nearly 3 million views

Voted San Diego's Best Personal Trainer 2010 and 2011 by The San Diego Union Tribune

Nutrition advisor for the Cardiovascular Disease Foundation

Trainer to the Trainers: Expert contributor to many national publications, including *Muscle & Fitness*, as well as former columnist for the NSCA's *Performance Training Journal*

www.ingramcontent.com/pod-product-compliance
Lightning Source LLC
Chambersburg PA
CBHW060840280326
41934CB00007B/860